The Life of the Skin

The
Life of the Skin

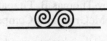

Arthur K. Balin, M.D., Ph.D.
Loretta Pratt Balin, M.D.

and

Marietta Whittlesey

Foreword by Albert M. Kligman, M.D., Ph.D.

Bantam Books
New York • Toronto • London • Sydney • Auckland

THE LIFE OF THE SKIN

A Bantam Book

Grateful acknowledgment is made for permission
to reprint from *Dermatology in General
Medicine* by Thomas B. Fitzpatrick, 1987,
The McGraw-Hill Companies.

Copyright © 1997 by Arthur K. Balin, M.D., Ph.D., Loretta Pratt
Balin, M.D., and Marietta Whittlesey.
Foreword copyright © 1997 by Albert M. Kligman, M.D., Ph.D.
Book design by James Sinclair.

ISBN 0-553-09719-9

PRINTED IN THE UNITED STATES OF AMERICA

We dedicate this book to the late D. Martin Carter, M.D., Ph.D., who inspired everyone around him, patients and doctors alike, to be the best they could be.

CONTENTS

ACKNOWLEDGMENTS

Any book is, to some degree, a group effort. Our special thanks go to the following individuals who were important to this book: our agents, Herb and Nancy Katz, whose energy and vision are on every page. Our editor, Toni Burbank, who was clear-eyed and a pleasure to work with, and her assistant, Adrienne Chew, who kept things running smoothly. Pam Luttrell and Virginia Corcoran at the offices of Drs. Balin and Pratt went out of their way to be helpful. Dr. Benjamin Balin, Sally Kirsner Balin, and Doreen Pratt all gave the kind of special thought, support, and love that only parents can give. Lynn Webb once again gave her valuable assistance in the whole project. Special thanks to Nellie Sabin and Addison Berkey for their good advice and constant support.

In addition, we would like to thank all of the patients and others who agreed to be interviewed for this book. While identifying characteristics of each patient have been changed, each patient in these stories is based on a particular patient or is a composite of more than one.

FOREWORD

Albert M. Kligman, M.D., Ph.D.

Back when I began, the field of dermatology was a swamp of snakes and nonsense, magic and folklore. The cynical view used to be that people went into dermatology so they didn't have to be awakened at night to go care for patients. In my day dermatologists were not even considered doctors.

But over the last decade the field has been transformed. Modern dermatology is rooted in science and developing at an Olympic pace. These days the highest-ranking students apply for dermatology residencies. To become a dermatologist now, a student has to be highly educated and conversant in the fields of psychology, art, immunology, genetics, and biochemistry, to name but a few. The changes are so rapid and so spectacular, I only wish I were not eighty years old so that I could be around to see what will be going on in dermatology in another twenty years.

Dr. Arthur Balin and Dr. Loretta Pratt are an unusual team of dermatologists. They are both at home in the fascinating, complex playground of the skin. They are married and they practice together—happily, as is clear from this account.

This is not the sort of book one might expect from Arthur Balin, with his impressive scholarly background, his six board certifications, and his international reputation in the field of aging research. This is an intimate, personal, and mainly optimistic account of the challenges and joys, doubts and dilemmas of two practicing dermatologists. I have been a dermatologist for fifty years, but I still feel invigorated and refreshed by the telling experiences and anecdotes in this delightful book, which although filled with cutting-edge science is also a love story. It is filled with the Balins' love of medicine and their love for their patients, their families, and each other.

What We Live For

—————◎⁄◎—————

Expectant mothers are fearful creatures. Their sleep is plagued by nightmares of monsters growing in their wombs; their daydreams conjure babies born with fatal diseases or missing limbs. My pregnancy was haunted by fears only a dermatologist could entertain. My imagination, of course, had plenty of fodder, for, during my medical training, I had attended babies born with skin diseases so terrible that even a missing limb might have seemed a lighter sentence. I had witnessed firsthand the pain and bewilderment of new parents who had thought of everything going wrong *but* their baby's skin. Most of these weren't problems that could be detected prenatally. And of those that can be diagnosed *in utero*, one doesn't test for them unless there is good reason to do so—not just to allay a nervous mother's fears. It's expensive, and they're too rare. Fortunately for most expectant mothers, their ignorance of most of these rare diseases prevents their entertaining such academic fears in the first place.

During my pregnancy, several of my patients had envied aloud my medical training. "I wish I'd been able to answer all my own questions during *my* pregnancy the way you must have been able to. Lucky you!" I wasn't so sure. In my case, being a doctor may actually have made me feel more helpless and even more fearful than the usual expectant mother, for I was hyperaware of the possibilities, of the "worst case scenarios" and "negative outcomes" (what universes of suffering are couched behind these clinical terms!). Whereas usually my medical training *did* give me an inner sense of competence and capability, my pregnancy put me on equal footing with every other expectant mother. I would just have to wait and see.

And so, when, after a long and exhausting birth, Arthur held our daughter for me to see, I scanned her skin anxiously.

"She looks like you, Arthur," I said at my first glimpse of our baby, who Arthur had known from the day we decided to get married would be a girl we would name Allison.

"I think she looks like a startled bunny rabbit," he replied, so uncharacteristically daffy with adoration that I stared at him. But then immediately the dermatologist took over. "Her skin is perfect," he pronounced. "Not even a stork bite [a particular blush at the back of a newborn's neck]. Nothing. Think how long it's been since we've seen skin like this."

I could barely wait to hold her, to touch her, to begin the lifelong dialogue in the language we all share, even with other mammals. The anthropologist Ashley Montagu, who has written so much about touch, calls it "the mother of the senses." It is the first to develop in fetal life and usually one of the last to depart in old age. As the nascent being comes to awareness, the senses switch on one by one, like lights coming on in the darkness. The earlier a function appears in embryogenesis, the more fundamental it is likely to be. The skin, the primary organ of touch, develops from the same embryonic layer as the brain. In fact, the sense of touch can pinch hit for other senses—perhaps most importantly, sight. Helen Keller spoke of not only reading and writing with her fingers but also of "remembering" in her fingers.

Babies do not come into the world *tabula rasa*. I knew that even before birth, Allison's skin had functioned as a nervous system, receiving and translating messages from my body and possibly even from the outer world. (Although developmental scientists do not presently believe the fetus can see or smell or taste before birth, there is increasing evidence that it can hear.) For most of her first nine months of life, she had been in nearly constant skin-to-skin communication with me. Tactile sensations of who knows what later significance had been constantly imprinting themselves. Infants join our world anticipating a continuation of the encasing pressure of the womb. We now know that the lips are the first area of the skin to come alive to touch during fetal life. Some fetuses can be observed to suck their thumbs and immediately resume this self-comforting or self-stimulating gesture after they are born. The lips are primed to begin seeking the mother's breast. For the newborn, touch is synonymous with survival.

At last, Allison was handed to me to hold. Gently I ran the tips of my fingers across her cheek. It registered against the skin of my own fingers as the softest thing I had ever stroked. No flower petal, no silk, no kid could match it. I breathed in her delicious scent, both yeasty and sweet, and I fell deeply and permanently in love. I found that tears were running down my cheeks, not only for the joy of those first few moments together but also because it was all so perfect—a clean slate. And she was so beautiful! This was it: the human skin in all its glory. This was Arthur's and my grail—perfect skin, unmarred by disease or the ravages of the environment or poor care.

How any but the most emotionally ill mother could not become addicted to touching and soothing her own baby I couldn't imagine, but as I began to bond with our daughter, I recalled the case of a little boy named Edward who spent some time in the pediatric department at Beth Israel during my medical school rotation there.

Edward was being worked up for what is called in medicine *failure to thrive*, a descriptive term meaning that a child isn't growing right. Maybe he's not gaining weight or length or height normally; maybe he's actually losing weight. In some cases, failure to thrive can be attributed to some sort of underlying disease—kidney failure, heart disease, a congenital disease like cystic fibrosis. But a heart-wrenching number, probably the majority, of these babies are failing to thrive not because of a disease, but because they aren't being handled and loved. This is not to say these children are necessarily outright abused, although some are. In general, these aren't the infants who come in with evidence of past fractures or the recognizable scars left by intentional injury. Nevertheless, they do have about them an air of deprivation and despair.

Edward was almost two years old and very small for his age. He was easily startled and cried inconsolably when surprised. When you looked him in the eye and smiled, he didn't return the gaze or smile back. In fact, he seemed completely uninterested in anything in his surroundings except a fuzzy sheep that one of the nurses had put in his crib. Bedtime was always a trial. He hated to be put to bed and, once tucked in, had unusual difficulty falling and staying asleep. One of the things I found most disturbing about his behavior was his proclivity to eat bizarre things, like dirt from the potted plants in the playroom, lint from the carpeting, or scraps of paper. This, coupled with his small size, led me to assume he was probably malnourished.

I remember seeing his mother a few times. She was a wan girl in her early twenties who seemed almost as dispirited as her child. What, I wondered, could be wrong with her that she didn't even notice her child wasn't growing until Edward was admitted to the hospital with epiglottitis, a life-threatening upper airway infection, and the admitting physician questioned the accuracy of Edward's age.

Later, I learned the story. Edward's mother, Lisa, was a single parent. Her boyfriend had departed the moment her pregnancy was evident, but her family had stood by her and supported their daughter and her baby so that both had food and shelter. From what we could gather, Edward had enough to eat, even though he had a picky appetite and seemed to take little pleasure in food. Eventually, when the results of Edward's endocrine studies came back relatively normal, his doctors turned to Lisa and delved into Edward's and her life together. What they discovered was a depressed, withdrawn girl who had barely enough energy to feed and dress her child and none left over to engage him in the sort of mother-infant communication essential to normal development. Their days, it seemed, were joyless and lonely. Amazingly, Lisa rarely touched her baby. There was none of the happy cuddling and cooing and playing that constitute the normal mother-child attachment. She really only handled him when she changed him or fed him. Most of the time, he lay alone in his crib staring at the ceiling or clutching a toy while Lisa slept or watched television in her bed in the hallway, wondering how such an enormous gulf had sprung up between herself and the rest of the world. Edward's growth problem actually stemmed from a lack of interaction, both psychological and tactile. Lisa's problem—and Edward's too— was chronic depression.

A wide array of human and animal studies have corroborated what normal mothers know: babies need to be cuddled and touched—a lot—in order to grow. Among the skin's many functions, it is the boundary between the inner self and the outside world. In a symposium on touch in infancy, Dr. Montagu said that for years he longed to give a lecture called "Radiology and Love." Although he did deliver the lecture many times, no medical school allowed him to use what they considered an extremely confusing title for his talk. The gist of the lecture was that people who have not been loved and handled during childhood show lines of retarded growth in the shinbone. X-rays of the fingers of neonates born to mothers who were emotionally disturbed during pregnancy likewise show specific radiologic abnormalities.

I later read a study by Dr. Tiffany Field at the Touch Research Institute at the University of Miami School of Medicine. She found that premature infants who were massaged gained weight nearly half again as fast as, and matured more rapidly than, those who were merely protected inside an incubator. Another study by Dr. Field and some of her colleagues showed that massage by itself was capable of increasing levels of serotonin, the same neurotransmitter that responds to the antidepressant Prozac. In the same experiment, it was discovered that massage also boosted the immune system by increasing the number and killing power of natural killer cells, a type of white blood cell that, among other effects, helps suppress burgeoning tumors. Massage was one of the first forms of medicine. Like many of the best medicines, it allows the body to heal itself. We now know that stimulating the skin causes the release of growth factors and hormones and probably of other substances that act on the central nervous system.

I wish I could say Lisa and Edward had been enrolled in one of Dr. Fields's studies that used massage to help treat depressed teenage mothers and neglected infants. However, their story, as long as I was able to follow it, gave every appearance of ending well. Lisa was introduced to a parenting group at the hospital, where she was able to get much-needed support and advice about caring for her child. I believe she had a brief course of antidepressant therapy and was hooked up with a social worker who could help her negotiate her way into a life that worked for herself and her baby.

Whenever I think of the urgency of the human need for touch and its importance to humankind, I am reminded of the part of the Sistine Chapel ceiling that shows God's finger bringing the divine spark to Adam. Across that small synapse, between the skin of one person's hand and that of another, travels as much meaning as is contained in all the books of the world—travels the essence of life.

Mothers have understood the deep importance of touching their children since the first mother caressed her infant or swaddled him in cloth while she returned to work in the fields. Medical science, however, is just beginning to corroborate this traditional mother wit in its clumsy attempt to quantify and provide a rationale for the importance of touch in human development and the maintenance of emotional health.

I can remember, during my medical school rotation in the neonatal intensive care unit, signs on the babies' incubators that said, chillingly, "Do not touch unnecessarily." At that point, majority medical opinion held that these premature infants were too fragile to touch. We had seemingly forgotten that they had come from a universe where their skin was constantly caressed by the walls of the uterus and bathed in a warm amniotic sea of constant temperature, constant darkness. At birth they lose their fleshy swaddling, their soothing waters, and are thrust headfirst, usually, into a harsh world of dry air, blinding light, alien sounds. And yet for so long, we neglected to replace these comforts with the smell and touch of a mother, or at least the solace of warm, skin-to-skin contact. Clearly, our children come to our world needing to be touched and spoken to through their skin. How we let them down by withholding the warmth of our bodies and the solace of our touch! In fact, even the tiniest preemies are well prepared in the womb to meet us. Their skin is not too fragile for loving handling. Babies are born with skin that already functions almost as it will in later life. Although thinner and more fragile than it will be in a few months, it is still a sturdy fabric, capable of performing most of the mature skin's array of functions.

During the months of my pregnancy, I used to dream about the little being forming inside me and preparing for life in another world. Naturally, some of my dreams were a skin doctor's dreams. I knew that by a few weeks after her conception, she was already encased in her own protective sheathing, called the *stratum corneum.* This horny layer of dead skin cells forms a watertight barrier that saves us from becoming either desiccated or water-logged. Later in my pregnancy, I marked the time when Allison's sebaceous glands began to function. They would soon be producing the *vernix caseosa,* the cheeselike mantle surrounding the newborn at birth. I wondered how she would smell. Mothers and babies can actually recognize each other's unique scent. Our individual scent is due to sebaceous gland secretions in the skin.

I thought about how vulnerable she would be, how naked to the light: what infant skin *does* lack for the first several months of life is any ability to protect itself in the sun. This is because a new-born's supply of melanin, the pigment that protects against sun-burn and largely determines skin color, is in shorter supply at birth than later. The morning after our baby was born, Arthur and I went to visit her in the nursery. Next to Allison's crib, a tiny black infant lay in hers. Even at birth, the pigment in her skin stood ready to protect her from a stronger sun. Would she better withstand the searing sunlight of the twenty-first century, a world in which the depletion of the earth's protective ozone layer might make half an hour in the sun the equivalent of half a day in today's atmosphere? Could Arthur and I protect our little girl? In a world where deadly skin cancers were increasing every year, could our cautions keep Allison safe?

"It's too bad babies can't wear sunscreen," Arthur said, tuning in, as he so often does, to my unspoken thoughts. Because the infant's skin doesn't function well as a barrier for several months, substances applied to a baby's skin are easily absorbed through the skin and into the bloodstream.

"And then she's going to wear it every single minute!" I replied. "I know I can keep her skin perfect like this forever. If she doesn't get sunburned and doesn't smoke . . . oh, if only she'll listen!" Was this roiling vehemence just postpartum hormones, or was I always going to worry about our child's skin? Was I always going to see her through a doctor's eyes?

As it turned out, I did continue to worry. Although I was fortunate in that my mother cared for Allison after I returned to work, she had raised me in an era when mothers were advised to send children out to play in the sun, and I was never quite sure I had my mother entirely convinced of what I knew to be right.

One sunny day after I had been back at work for a few months, I had one of those scary flashes of maternal intuition. I was overcome with the certainty that my mother had forgotten to put Allison's sunblock and sun hat on her. To me, this was akin to letting her play with matches or play unattended near the pool. Leaving a patient prepped on the table for a facial peel, I rushed to call home. Sure enough, I had been correct.

"Oh Loretta, oh dear, I was going to call you," my mother said before I could even ask about the sunscreen. "You're going to be so upset. I forgot Allison's sunscreen and her sun hat when we went out for our walk, and she's a little red."

"Oh Mom, how *could* you? It's the one thing I've begged you to be careful about! She's going to have wrinkles when she's thirty because of this day. You won't listen to me about your own skin, but I won't let you ruin hers." My sister later told me she thought I had overreacted, but it's been shown repeatedly that nearly all the sun damage that will lead to wrinkles and skin cancers in later life has occurred by age eighteen.

"I'm so sorry, Loretta. I can't believe I forgot. She had a bad morning after you left, and I took her out in her carriage to calm her down, and I just forgot. What should I do? Is there anything I can put on her face?"

"No. There's nothing you can do. I'm coming home as soon as I finish with my next patient." I was seething. I buzzed Arthur to inform him of the disaster, but he was doing surgery and couldn't come to the phone. I thought about going upstairs to see him, but then I remembered my patient waiting to have her face peeled.

As I swabbed the acid onto my patient's face, I began to calm down. The face in front of me had fairly severe sun damage—grooves on the upper lip and forehead, liver spots, the overall pouchy sallowness of badly treated skin approaching middle age—

but after all, it had taken many years of careless exposure to get it that way. I thought of my poor mother sitting there with my words still stinging her ears. She's very sensitive, and I felt guilty about my outburst. I knew this wouldn't be the last time Allison was exposed to the sun without protection. Even Arthur once forgot his sunblock while sailing and came home sheepish and red. It was just that this was the first encroachment into the perfection of her skin. I knew I couldn't protect her from getting earaches or colds or maybe even breaking her leg skiing with her father. But I had considered her skin my domain, and one I could control. My attention now really could prevent everything from wrinkles to skin cancer later in Allison's life.

As soon as I had finished with my patient, I called my mother back and apologized.

"Oh Loretta, I'll never let it happen again," she choked.

And she hasn't. But for most of Allison's first year, I would call my mother from the office every sunny morning before she got Allison dressed to remind her about the sun protection.

I look forward to the day when I can teach Allison herself about protecting her skin. I imagine one of her sixteenth-birthday presents will be a tube of Retin-A to protect her against skin cancers—unless there's something even better by then. Sam, Arthur's son by his first marriage, learned about his skin early. I remember one day when Sam was about six and was walking with Arthur and me along a beach crowded with sunbathers he suddenly began to tug at Arthur's hand. "Daddy, Daddy," he exclaimed. "You'd better go tell those people they're going to get skin cancer!"

Sometimes in those early months after I myself had caught a little sleep, I would sit by Allison's crib, gazing at her, exactly as I had seen so many other enraptured new mothers doing. As she lay sleeping, her tiny fists curled into tight little shells, her orbits following who could imagine what dreams behind translucent eyelids, I had time to ponder motherhood and medicine. There can be a certain level of frustration in caring for patients, because of the limitations of the doctor-patient relationship. One obviously can't take patients home and nurture them, yet in some cases, that sort of all-encompassing care is what's really needed. Motherhood was my chance to apply my entire being to the protection and education and nurture of another person. It filled in an even more complete way a deep instinct and need to heal and protect that had led me to become a doctor and to choose dermatology.

I fell in love with dermatology. I was later surprised to learn that some people assume doctors choose dermatology as a specialty just because there aren't usually emergencies and unpredictable hours or because they think we can charge a lot to do procedures, particularly cosmetic ones. But none of those reasons entered my thinking at the time I chose dermatology as my life's work. In fact, it wasn't a decision I made with my mind so much as with my heart. I fell in love with dermatology during my first week in that department during medical school. I knew immediately that I had found my calling. Part of what I loved was that it was so visual. Skin disease is visually apparent, and later, when I have successfully treated a patient, I can see what I have done. The cystic acne is gone, the sun damage is gone, the pretty, hopeful face beneath is restored.

Dermatology is highly tactile as well. Sometimes the simple feel of a skin lesion tells us all we need to know, without any fancy diagnostic tests. Often, for instance, one can't see a precancerous skin lesion, but in lightly feeling a patient's skin, one's fingertips immediately detect areas that feel like sandpaper. Other skin lesions are distinguished by their firmness or by dimpling that appears if the area is pressed. Touching is often the best way to monitor improvement like skin softening in response to medication.

I think there are many misconceptions about dermatologists, and I shared them until those first days of my dermatology rotation. In reality, dermatologists do far more than treat the skin, for the skin mirrors the health of the entire body. Besides answering my need to restore my patients' appearance, it was a specialty in which I could apply every bit of medical knowledge I had learned. So often a skin eruption or color change is the first sign of something else going wrong in the deeper organs. The alert dermatologist can diagnose lupus and sarcoidosis and many types of cancer, to name only a few problems. The work is hardly just skin deep.

Then, of course, there was the burgeoning field of aging research. I was doing my medical training at a time when enormous advances were being made in the areas of cutaneous rejuvenation. Retin-A was being studied, various techniques of facial peeling were coming to the fore. People were realizing that the visual stigmata of aging were abnormal and could be prevented or reversed. Even before I met Arthur Balin, this area of dermatology beckoned to me, because again it permitted me to do more than make people well. It gave me the chance to make them happy too.

When, as a fourth-year medical student, I first encountered Arthur, he was already a renowned clinician and investigator in the field of aging research. Although Arthur claims he doesn't remember meeting me that day, it was he who showed me around the Laboratory of Investigative Dermatology he and his colleagues from Yale were in the process of building at Rockefeller University in New York City. I still had my internship year ahead of me, but I was hoping to do my residency at Cornell–New York Hospital, which would also mean I would be connected with Arthur's group next door at Rockefeller.

I was quite intimidated by Arthur that day, because he didn't say very much. He was already legendary; maybe he couldn't be bothered with such a neophyte as myself. Knowing him as I do now, I realize it was probably he who was the more intimidated. Arthur is one of the shyest people I have ever met. Yet his patients invariably find him solicitous and interested in their lives. Standing outside the door when Arthur is removing a skin cancer or performing liposuction, one hears the classical music he always plays when he is working, and a more or less steady stream of conversation. He becomes voluble when he is with patients, because he cares about putting frightened people at their ease. But small talk does not come easily to him. Try chit-chatting with him when he is back in his own world, and the conversation quickly dies—as it did much of that day he was showing me the impressive facility they were building. I later mentioned him to a friend of mine from med school who was doing a dermatology residency at Yale, where Arthur had just come from, and he said, "That guy's a genius. He'll probably win a Nobel. If anyone can figure out how to make us live forever, Arthur Balin can do it. He's nice, too. He's not chatty, and even though he probably doesn't know who Mick Jagger is, he's a real person. The other thing about Dr. Balin is that deep in there, there's a great sense of humor just dying to get out."

Then, as now, Arthur's interests lay in basic research into the life span of cells. Except for cancer cells, mammalian cells are not immortal. They have a finite capacity for division. Then something turns them off, and they cannot divide anymore. What it is that switches off was the subject of part of Arthur's basic quest, although along the way, he learned things about cell growth that had important clinical applications. As I spent time around the lab, I was sure my friend was right: if anyone could discover the fountain of youth, it was Arthur Balin.

Now, looking down at our little girl at the beginning of her life, I hoped with all my heart that her father might one day discover how to help her live to be well beyond one hundred years. Perhaps his research into the mysteries of cellular life span might help us learn how to defeat the immortality of cancer cells. I would be right there working alongside him, learning everything I could about how to make her life wonderful. All this had a closure that felt right. With her arrival, the research wasn't just theoretical. Our scientific goals and our parental goals had merged into an even more urgent one—that of ensuring the quality of Allison's life.

The Skin Is the Hero

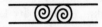

"Two layers compose the skin—the superficial epidermis and, deeper, the dermis. Between is a plane of pure energy where the life-force is in full gallop."

RICHARD SELZER, M.D.
MORTAL LESSONS: NOTES ON THE ART OF SURGERY

Once, when I was a young boy, I heard a gruesome story that changed forever my view of my skin. Perhaps it was this early imprint that impressed me with the notion of our skin as a precious, life-preserving tissue we must do our best to protect. The story concerned a child circus performer. Probably the story impressed me at the time because he was a boy of my own age. In order to costume him for a new act, the circus spray-painted his entire body with gold paint. Several hours later, he was dead. Unable to disperse the heat of his life processes, the boy had literally cooked to death inside his own skin, his rising body temperature having destroyed the hundreds of enzymes necessary for life. For among the many essential functions of our skin is temperature regulation.

For all I know, this story is apocryphal. But it was my earliest understanding that, far from being an inert rind, our skin is as essential for life as our brain and our other organs. I know that many of my patients come in thinking of their skin as little more than a decorative sausage casing and skin diseases as largely cosmetic problems. Nothing is further from the truth. Our skin is the most important interface between our inner universe and the outer

· 13 ·

world. We are identified largely by our skin—its color, hairiness, the way it drapes over our features. Our hair, which is really an extension of our skin, contributes significantly to our appearance. The skin and hair are both key organs of sexual attraction and fulfillment. The human skin is also part DEW line, part laboratory, part switchboard, and part thermostat. In constant communication with our brain, our skin contributes an essential part of our intelligence. It is our largest sensory organ and arguably our most important one, for while other sensory organs are clustered in a small area at the front of our face, the skin sensors are on every millimeter of our skin. In this way, the skin tells us what we feel—not only the sensations of things contacting our skin but also where our bodies are in three-dimensional space at any moment.

When I meet a new patient for the first time, I do not know how deep into his or her skin I will need to see. If you were to come to my office for a consultation, I would start by examining your skin at the lowest magnification I use—with my naked eyes, aided only by my eyeglasses. From a social distance, all I survey with my eyes is dead. Human beings are actually encased in a seamless raincoat of dead cells known as the stratum corneum. Your stratum corneum represents the final stage in the life cycle of the cells that make up your epidermis, or outer layer of skin. The life cycle of epidermal cells begins at the interface between the epidermis and the dermis, the next layer down. It is both a temporal and a spatial progression. During the twenty-eight or so days required to complete the cycle, cells are born at the lowest layer and migrate upward to the surface. As they make their way toward the light, they synthesize filaments of a waxy, waterproof protein called *keratin.* By the time the cells reach the upper layer of your skin, where their task is to form a protective barrier to the outside world, they have become clogged with this cellular armor. A complex network of these dead keratinized cells "glued" together forms our protective sheathing. In death, they repose on our surfaces, protecting the living human universe within. But they, too, are continually being shed and replaced by newer generations of dead cells.

Despite being encased in the cutaneous equivalent of canvas, your epidermis feels soft and pliable—rather than cornified, like the shell of a turtle or armadillo—because it is coated with a thin layer of a fatty, oily substance called *sebum.* This sebum-coated outer layer of skin protects us from physical insults, keeps vital fluids inside, and prevents our becoming waterlogged from the outside. The waterproof stratum corneum is only one-hundredth of a millimeter thick, but it is all that stands between you and a fatal mingling with the outer environment.

In addition to its role as the body's sheathing, the epidermis is now known to be a major front in the immune system. *Langerhans cells,* studded throughout the epidermis, recognize foreign substances and present them to other immune-system cells in the blood, which then mount an appropriate campaign against them. Langerhans cells are an important first line of defense against environmental invaders. It seems fitting that the organ that defines the boundary between outside and inside worlds would be involved in the essential immune-system task of distinguishing between self and other. The human body is actually a thesaurus of such metaphors.

The epidermis, like the liver, is also part chemical plant. In addition to synthesizing vitamin D in the presence of sunlight, the skin is capable of modifying a variety of chemical compounds that contact it. The epidermis can also chemically inactivate dangerous substances that could otherwise be absorbed through the skin.

Still maintaining my social distance from you as we sit face to face in my office, I notice your skin color. The difference among the races is arguably due most prominently to differences in skin color or pigmentation. Yet try telling an ardent supporter of apartheid or other institutionalized racial segregation that skin color is the same for us all throughout most layers of our skin. The stratum corneum, if removed, has the same grayish, transparent look regardless of race. The dermis, the thicker layer below the epidermis, is the same shade in all of us. The differences, then, are determined by denizens of the lowest level of the epidermis, known as *melanocytes.* These cells produce the pigment *melanin,* which determines the intensity of your skin's and hair's color. There are two types of melanin, each a slightly different shade: *eumelanin,* which is blackish-brown, and *pheomelanin,* which is reddish-yellow. Most white people owe their skin color to eumelanin—only fair-skinned redheads make pheomelanin. The melanocytes manufacture one or the other type of melanin, according to one's genetic background. The difference in skin color between blacks and whites is actually due to the amount, type, and arrangement of the melanin within the epidermis, because each of us has the same number of melanocytes. Carotenes, which are mostly located a level deeper, in the dermis, lend the yellowish cast to Asian skins, while hemoglobin, the oxygen-carrying pigment in blood, lends pinkness to some fair skins. Albinos are genetically unable to produce any melanin at all. Their pinkish cast is due to hemoglobin unmixed with melanin. Aside from having caused hideous racial strife since the beginning of time, melanin's real purpose is to absorb ultraviolet light and protect us from sun damage not only to our skin but also to the DNA carried in all the cells of our bodies. In that sense, the darker your natural skin color, the more melanin you have and the better adapted you are to life under our sun.

Although, from a polite distance, the surface of your epidermis appears hairless and smooth, it is neither. We humans call ourselves "naked apes," yet we are far from nude. Even areas of your body that you suppose hairless are covered with fine, unpigmented hairs, often too small to be perceived by unamplified vision. Despite their near-invisibility, they are actually ultrasensitive touch sensors. We are the only mammals with such highly sensitive touch receptors all over our bodies. Our entire integument is as sensitive as an animal's whiskers, which are restricted to a small part of the face. It requires a brain as large as the human brain to process this constant sensory input from the skin. If every hair on, for example, a cat's body were as sensitive as its whiskers, the cat would need a much larger brain.

The epidermis has myriad textures. Think about the skin patterns and textures of such areas as your elbows, palms, and lips. Skin surface markings are especially developed on the friction surfaces of the hands and feet, where the epidermis is thickest. The patterns of alternating ridges and valleys of these areas are called *dermatoglyphics,* and we share these features only with other primates.

The best-known dermatoglyphics are fingerprints. They are formed during the third and fourth months of fetal life and remain unchanged throughout our lives. What is most astounding about these dermatoglyphics is the uniqueness of their patterns. Of the nearly two hundred million sets of fingerprints on file at the FBI, no identical sets have ever been discovered. Even identical twins, whose fingerprints may bear many gross resemblances to one another, still have subtle differences.

To take a closer look at your skin, I must put on magnifiers. With their aid, I can now see smaller surface markings not immediately apparent from a conversational distance. The majority of these are acquired spots and barnacles that accumulate in the epidermis with time and sun exposure. At this low magnification I can get a better view of your freckles, which are due to increased melanin production, and *solar lentigines,* the flat, brown "liver spots" arising from an abnormal increase in the number of melanin-producing cells, which clump together in spotty patches. I can see *nevocellular nevi,* or moles, caused by tightly packed groups of melanocytes, and *seborrheic keratoses,* which resemble moles, although not to the trained eye. Scaling pink or yellowish patches called *actinic,* or solar, keratoses—actually early-stage skin cancers—are also clear to me at this magnification, although I can often detect them just by running the tip of my forefinger over the skin and feeling their telltale sandpaper texture. Through my magnifiers, I can more easily see clusters of dilated blood vessels called *telangiectasias,* or "spider veins." These can be caused by chronic sun exposure and by the female hormone, estrogen. Spider veins may also herald liver disease. It is said that New York City barmaids of the nineteenth century referred to chronic inebriates among their clientele as "spiders" for this reason. One of the liver's many functions in both sexes is to break down female hormones. Compromised liver function may cause an increase in female hormones and, consequently, the appearance of spider veins and enlarged breasts in men.

A deeper view of your skin is available to me from the surface. Using a special ultraviolet-light camera, I can photograph your face and see its future already recorded deep within the epidermis. In my viewfinder, you may appear to my naked eye as a twenty-five-year-old with what some people might call a "good" tan scattered with a few freckles. But what the film reveals is a veritable Jackson Pollock painting of splashed and scattered blotches of melanin. Still hidden beneath the surface and invisible to the naked eye, perhaps for decades to come, it is the fallout of ultraviolet bombardment. Patients who insist they have done little damage to their skin are always amazed and horrified by what this special camera reveals of their future appearance!

If I needed to go deeper into your skin, I would remove some for a biopsy. If the biopsy were to come back positive for skin cancer, I might, depending upon the method of removal you chose, get a much deeper and detailed look into your skin. Examining a section of your skin under an optical microscope, I can see the tightly packed cells of the layers of the normal epidermis. If the epidermal cells are undergoing cancerous changes, the usual neat architecture of these rows of epidermal cells degenerates, and they become large and disorganized. Leaving the diaphanous mantle of the epidermis, my eye travels to the dermis, the next layer of skin, which gives structure, strength, and heft to the human integument and connects it to the blood supply and the nervous system. The underside of the epidermis and the top layer of the dermis form an interlocking mirror image of one another's surfaces.

The dermis is a cushiony matrix made up of *collagen* and *elastin* fibers embedded in an amorphous gel known as *ground substance*. The body contains at least eleven different types of collagen, each with a different structure and function. Bone, cartilage, and connective tissue all contain collagen. What they have in common is their structure: three separate chains of protein wound tightly around one another. The sequence and arrangement of these protein chains are what differentiate the types of collagen. Each three-chain arrangement makes up what is called a *fibril*. Collagen fibers, which look to the naked eye like wisps of fiberglass, are actually bundles of these tiny fibrils. Seen through a microscope, collagen appears as pink patches in the skin sections. To the much more powerful scanning electron microscope, collagen most resembles pipe cleaners. Cells in the dermis called *fibroblasts* synthesize collagen.

Woven in amongst the collagen fibers of the skin, like the warp and woof of the human fabric, are fibers of a pliable protein called elastin. Elastin—which, like collagen, can't be absorbed from expensive skin creams, all claims to the contrary—is capable of stretching like a rubber band and then snapping back to its original length. Collagen fibers lend tensile strength to the skin, while elastin gives it resilience, but although skin is flexible and can stretch to accommodate enormous weight gains or pregnancy, collagen fibers can be stretched to the point of tearing, leaving behind permanent stretch marks, or *striae.*

The blood vessels in the dermis can hold up to 25 percent of the body's blood supply at any one time. Any substance that can penetrate the epidermis and reach the dermis can enter the bloodstream through the dermis's rich vascular network. It is this ready interface of dermis and bloodstream that has permitted the engineering of transdermal drugs. When a drug-containing patch is placed on the skin, the active drug is combined with a substance that penetrates the epidermis and delivers the drug to the dermis, where it can be taken up into the circulation and dispersed throughout the body. This mode of delivery provides a steady, sustained release of hormones, like estrogen or testosterone, or nicotine or cancer chemotherapy drugs without their having to be injected, swallowed, or smoked.

Scattered throughout the dermis are several different types of glands: *sebaceous glands,* which produce sebum, and *eccrine sweat glands,* which are in the service of the body's temperature-regulating system. Although the hypothalamus in the brain is the body's mastermind of temperature regulation, the skin is its functionary. When we are in danger of overheating, our sweat glands pour out fluid that cools the skin as it evaporates. When we are cold, blood vessels in the dermis contract and shunt blood to our body core, which must stay within a narrow temperature range if we are to live.

Human skin contains two types of sweat glands. The *apocrine* sweat glands are found primarily in the underarms and perineum, although the breast is also considered an apocrine gland. Apocrine glands are attached to hair follicles, into which the glands' ducts empty. These glands don't come into play until just before puberty. They are the odor-producing sweat glands that are the target of underarm deodorants. Most authorities believe that apocrine sweat gland secretions have no intrinsic odor and that the characteristic stench of underarm perspiration is due to bacterial action. This is the reason most deodorants contain antimicrobial agents.

The eccrine sweat glands are located on hairless areas of the skin, and their ducts open directly onto the skin surface. They produce a watery, cooling sweat. Interestingly, all right-handed people, and nearly all left-handed ones, produce more sweat on one side of the body than the other, usually on the side opposite the dominant hand.

I can see, even from looking at the surface of your skin, something about the activity of your oil-producing glands, the sebaceous glands. Oiliness, old acne scars, and soft skin despite advanced age all bespeak active sebaceous glands. Sebaceous glands are attached to hair follicles. In addition to keeping our skin and hair lubricated, sebum is the secretion to which each of us owes our unique scent. Sebaceous glands are influenced by male hormones and, until puberty, are small and limited in their effusions. That nemesis of adolescence, acne, is an inflammation and blockage of the sebaceous glands. As we age, we produce less sebum, which means an eventual end to acne for most people, but also drier, less waterproof skin. We have some instruments in our office that measures the skin's oil content, moisture level, ability to retain moisture, and several other features that permit us to assess your skin's physiologic functions. The skin's nerve network is housed in the upper dermis.

The skin is by far the largest sensory organ, and the processing of its sensory impulses occupies a large part of the cerebral cortex. An enormous share of all that we experience in the world comes to us through our skin. Not only does it swathe us in touch sensations—unique amalgams of hot, cold, sharp, soft, gentle, rough, smooth—the sense of touch is also an essential component of physical and psychic growth and development in humans and animals. Nerve receptors surrounding hair follicles and connecting them to the epidermis are probably the most important touch sensors. They are constantly in action, informing us about our surroundings. Although we are more aware of input from our eyes, ears, taste buds, and nose, these invisible antennae bristling from the surface of our skin can detect movements in air currents and other minuscule input and, in their constant interface with the brain, provide a steady stream of subliminal information about where we are located, the environment around us, and who is there with us. Without your even seeing or hearing it, you may sense that someone has quietly entered the room. Your sense of touch is what has just informed you that the air currents in the room have changed slightly and have brushed these innervated hairs. Even though the top layer of skin that we see is dead, the skin itself is extremely alive.

In addition to these receptors connected to hairs, *Meissner's corpuscles* lie at the dermal-epidermal junction on the palms and soles of primates, including humans. The *Vater-Pacini corpuscles* are deeper in the dermis. They are most numerous in the clitoris and fingers and are thought to perceive deep pressure. *Merkel's disks* lie at the top layers of the living part of the epidermis and are believed to relay sensations of continuous pressure.

If I am looking under the microscope at a section of skin from a hairy part of the body, I can see individual hair shafts scattered here and there in the dermis. At this magnification, they resemble the antennae of horseshoe crabs poking up from a beach. Hair develops from follicles embedded in the dermis. It is actually a column of dead, keratinized cells like those of the stratum corneum. Its primary function in many areas of the body is protection. Body hair is also an important sensory appendage in humans, although we are far outclassed in this respect by cats and dogs. The long hairs of the scalp, however, serve no discernible function beyond protection of the scalp from sun. In both sexes, their growth is controlled by sex hormones, which suggests that their main function may relate to sexual attraction and mating. Certainly this decorative and protective protein has, from the time of Samson, played a symbolic role in the human psyche. "The hair or hair-do is halfway between nature and culture, between skin and clothes, an ornament which delimits something visible and something hidden," writes Dr. Pomey Rey in his book *Skin and Psychology.* As such, the hair plays a major role in nonverbal communication. When men are surveyed as to what they notice first in a woman, hair always ranks high on the list.

The wondrous coat of many colors we call the skin is the heaviest organ of the human body, though not, as commonly believed, the largest. With regard to surface area, that distinction goes to the digestive tract. Skin covers an average of eighteen square feet and weighs about five pounds. Except when it is misbehaving during adolescence or tattling on us for our excesses or belying our age, many of us give our skin little thought beyond its daily wash or shave. Our hope is that the stories in this book will serve to acquaint more people with this miraculous web and permit them to understand more about this flag they fly in the world.

The skin itself has been the hero of this chapter, but the true heroes of this book are our patients. The clinical tales that follow contain stories of our patients—or people very much like our patients—who have come to us over the years for healing and transformation. It is also the story of our own transformation from medical student and researcher to wife and husband and finally to mother and father.

Written on the Skin

In the physiologic division of labor, it is often delegated to the skin to carry messages from the deeper organs. The health of the skin mirrors that of the rest of the body. Doctors learn that cutaneous symptoms like itching, color changes, unusual hair growth, and nail anomalies frequently herald the presence of visceral disease or disordered metabolism. The average person is aware that excessive pallor may mean anemia and that yellowness, or jaundice, indicates liver disease, while blueness, or cyanosis of the skin, means that the blood and tissues are starved for oxygen. The cutaneous harbingers of internal disease are legion. The yellow fingernails of chronic edema, the clubbed fingertips of lung disease, the downy facial hair of ovarian tumors are but a few. While the underlying disease may still be cloaked in silence deep within the body, the skin above can be sounding a clamorous alarm. In some instances, the skin may signal so vociferously as to develop a symptom directly over the site of a diseased internal organ, as in the case of a seventy-four-year-old woman who developed a port wine stain on her left breast—a breast that later was found to harbor a cancerous tumor. Other skin signs are quite specific markers for internal diseases, like the eruption known as *necrolytic migratory erythema,* which announces a specific type of pancreatic tumor. All physicians are taught to be mindful of these skin signs, which are, nonetheless, often disregarded as isolated, skin-deep phenomena. Early diagnoses of internal diseases are thereby missed.

Dermatologists are like fingerprint analysts in the crime lab of disease. If the skin is properly read, it may be found to reflect changes occurring at the cellular level in diseased organs. Its easy accessibility makes it ideal for taking samples that may provide clues to systemic diseases. So much of the skin doctor's art lies in understanding what is occurring beneath the surface. The alert dermatologist can often detect and diagnose internal diseases long before they are apparent even to the patient.

Perhaps nowhere can the skin tell a story better than in the dead, and its testimony is highly valued by pathologists and forensics experts. There is the mottling, known as *livor mortis,* which occurs as blood settles and helps determine the time of death. The condition of the skin bears everlasting witness to the means of death—the burns, bruises, strangulation marks, the cherry-red skin of carbon monoxide poisoning. Epidermal ridges, known as fingerprints, identify perpetrators beyond the shadow of a doubt. Many criminals owe their eventual capture to their ignorance of the skin's ability to tell a story and to tell it accurately.

During the years we were at Rockefeller we had as an important member of our team a technician named Ingrid Soderholm. It was Ingrid's job to grow cells in culture flasks for Arthur's various experiments. Ingrid had been born in a small town outside of Stockholm, had come to America to go to college, and had married a Swedish architect who practiced in New York.

Several years ago, Ingrid found herself caught up in the sort of medical nightmare that everyone dreads. Throughout the ordeal, her skin was telegraphing with all its usual clarity, yet the urgency of its message was eclipsed by the stronger signals issuing from other organs.

One day I arrived in the office about noon, having spent the morning making my weekly rounds at a nearby nursing home. It was a scalding July day, and many of the residents were suffering from bacterial skin infections encouraged by the warm, moist air at the nursing home. I was running behind schedule, and a patient was already waiting in one of my examining rooms. Nevertheless, I decided to take two minutes to check in with Arthur. I found him downstairs in the office from which he directs the American Aging Association and publishes the research journal *Age.* At my approach he swiveled around in his chair.

"We had a call from Ingrid. She's got some sort of medical problem, and she wants to come talk to us as soon as possible." He handed me a telephone number. It wasn't her lab number, and that in itself was unusual. Ingrid was exceptionally fit and healthy and prided herself on never missing a day of work.

"Do you know what it's about?"

"She didn't want to talk about it on the telephone."

As soon as I had a pause between patients I called Ingrid who was at home.

"Dr. Pratt," she said in a strained voice so unlike her normally ebullient self, "I hate to bother you, but I need some advice. I was wondering if I could take you out to lunch?"

"Of course we could have lunch," I said. "The only problem is that it will be a few weeks before I can get a day off to go to the city. Can this wait that long?"

"I don't really want to talk about it on the telephone, and I'd like to see you soon, but I know how busy you two are. My plan was to go down and spend the night with a friend in Delaware and meet you. I could just bring a sandwich to your office if you wanted."

Ingrid and I agreed to meet at a quiet restaurant near Arthur's and my office in three days. I hung up feeling alarmed and sad. Ingrid had been such an important part of Arthur's and my life for so long.

Ingrid was already waiting when I arrived. As usual, she looked the very picture of Nordic good health, her blond hair only slightly graying, her skin lovely as ever.

"Ingrid," I said. "I've been so worried since your call. Let's get right down to it. What's wrong?"

"Oh, Dr. Pratt," she said, "very, very bad news."

My heart jolted.

"For the last couple of months I've been having a little bit of chest pain and a dry cough that kept hanging around. Finally I decided to go have a chest x-ray. So I went, and I got the results back." She looked away, and her shoulders began to shake. I put my hand on her shoulder.

"They found several tumors in my lung, and they found metastases in the liver and colon."

My first reaction was disbelief. "Wait a minute. Something is wrong." For while it's true that some patients with metastatic lung cancer remain relatively asymptomatic until quite late in the course of their disease, there are usually signs—wheezing, a productive cough, weight loss, fatigue, a propensity to develop pneumonia and other respiratory infections. There had been none of that, and furthermore, Ingrid had never been a smoker. Although occasionally someone who has never smoked will develop lung cancer, 70 percent of lung cancers that arise in women are smoking-related. The whole situation felt terribly wrong. Or was it just that the idea of Ingrid's being mortally ill was too devastating to consider?

"All right," I said. "First we need a second opinion. This just doesn't ring true to me. I want you to come back to the office with me, and I'll get the phone number of a pulmonologist who is an old friend of Arthur's from Yale. He practices in Philadelphia, and he's very good. His name is Morty Bierman."

Ingrid nodded. "I will definitely go see him, but the other doctor seemed so positive. When I tried to tell him that I'd have to schedule any treatments around my job, he said, 'Don't bother. Quit your job and get your affairs in order. I don't think you can count on much time.' That's what he said. Just like that. Can you imagine? I thought to myself, 'I know Dr. Pratt and Dr. Balin would never treat a patient like that.' So I decided to come down and see you."

"When we get back to the office, you can give me the other doctor's phone number. I would like to see his report and I'm sure Arthur will want to as well," I said.

"Well," she said. "Let's talk about other things. I want to hear all about your new baby boy and Allison, who must be ready to start medical school herself, the little angel." And so she steered me away from her own problems, and I found myself telling her about our family and our research plans and the new facility we were building, but inside my mind was tumbling.

"I shouldn't necessarily be saying this," I blurted out in response to a question about my mother. "But I just have a gut feeling something is wrong here. You really need to see Dr. Bierman for his opinion. And Ingrid—even if the diagnosis is correct, Arthur and I will do everything we can to help you get the best treatment. We'll be right with you." I turned abruptly and pretended to be jotting down a note so that she wouldn't notice the tears pricking at my eyes. "I guess I'd better get back to my patients," I said. "Why don't you follow me in your car?" As I turned to put my wallet back in my purse, my eyes alighted briefly, almost unconsciously, on a small spot on Ingrid's upper arm. At that point, I merely noted it and kept on going, my mind already preparing itself for the long afternoon of patients in front of me.

I found it difficult to keep my mind on my patients that afternoon. Ingrid's anguished face kept floating before my mind's eye. Even doctors who work daily with terminally ill patients never fully come to terms with incurable disease and death.

Two days later, we received a faxed copy of the other physician's report. It read, "Chest x-ray revealed widespread pulmonary nodules especially in the right lower lobe. Chest CT revealed widespread pulmonary metastases, right hilar adenopathy and a right lower lobe conglomerative mass. Abdominal and pelvic CT revealed liver metastases, retroperitoneal adenopathy, bilateral hydronephrosis with calculi at the level of the left renal pelvis and abnormal thickening of the rectum." Under the paragraph titled *Assessment* he had written, "This is a well-nourished middle-aged black female with an unremarkable medical history, except for an episode of renal colic concomitant with renal calculi in 1993. She now appears to have a primary pulmonary malignancy with multiple metastases. Her possible diagnosis, need for further evaluation and staging were discussed with her."

Translated, this means, "This woman's chest x-rays showed many masses in the lungs, particularly in the bottom of the right lung. A computerized tomography (CT) scan of the lungs showed enlarged lymph nodes and cancer throughout her lungs. CT scans of the stomach and pelvis showed metastases to the liver, obstruction and atrophy of both kidneys, with a kidney stone on the left side, and an abnormality of the rectum that also suggests cancer. This patient has always been healthy except for a bout with kidney stones a few years ago. She now seems to have lung cancer that has spread all over her body." There was a glaring error in the first line of the assessment. To mistake Ingrid for a well-nourished, middle-aged black woman would have to be called a significant oversight, since Ingrid is a well-nourished, sixty-year-old *white* woman. A few paragraphs farther down, in the summary, Ingrid was correctly described. The date on the letter was a year off, I noticed. Details perhaps, but were they nonetheless indicative of a sloppy approach? So far, I was not impressed. In fact, I was enraged.

I thought about the situation as I ate supper with our daughter. Allison, then just fourteen months old, kept practicing her newest word, among the first she had spoken. *"Mole!"* she repeated emphatically, pointing to miscellaneous specks on my arms.

I didn't sleep well that night. As I lay there, turning from side to side in the humid July night, I kept thinking about Ingrid—how she had looked that afternoon sitting at the lunch table. I felt unusually restless. "Mole!" Allison kept insisting inside my head. "Mole!" Finally the cacophony propelled me out of bed. Arthur was still across the driveway, working in our medical library. I turned on the light.

I thought about how the field of molecular biology was exploding with new ideas and new information. We were learning so much about the genesis and physiology of cancer cells. There were the recently discovered tumor suppressor genes. There were enzyme systems capable of repairing damage to DNA before the alterations become part of the cell's instructions and caused it to become malignant. There was so much raw knowledge and still so few ways of applying it to help people with cancer. People like Ingrid.

I don't know whether it was Allison's voice chanting "mole" in my ear all evening or a moment of grace, but suddenly a possible answer dropped fully formed into my mind. The mark I had seen on Ingrid's upper arm that afternoon wasn't actually a mole. Every mark on the skin has a name, but the names, though abundantly descriptive as to color, texture, shape, and composition, do not constitute a diagnosis. Skin lesions can be macules, papules, plaques, nodules, vesicles, bullae, blebs, or pustules, to name but a few. Their color can be erythematous (red), violaceous, blue, or pearly. They can be round, oval, or linear. The pattern they make on the skin can be annular (ringlike) or linear, herpetiform (like a herpes eruption) or arciform (crescent-shaped). Their consistency can be doughy or firm, crusty, dry or moist. In one chapter of his classic textbook on dermatology, *Dermatology in General Medicine,* Thomas B. Fitzpatrick notes,

> Physicians must learn to "read" the skin as well as they are able to read an X-ray of the chest or interpret an electrocardiogram. . . . The individual lesions are analogous to the letters of the alphabet, and groups of lesions may be analogous to words or phrases. . . . To read words, one must recognize letters, to read the skin one must recognize the basic lesions. To understand a paragraph, one must know how words are put together; to arrive at a differential diagnosis, one must know what the basic lesions represent.

As I remembered it that midnight, Ingrid's spot was a small, flat, violaceous plaque. That in itself was unremarkable and wouldn't have led me anywhere. It was the confluence of signs—the skin lesion, the kidney stones, and the lung tumors—that spoke loudest. The fact that Ingrid was a Scandinavian further fortified my suspicions. Another disease provided a far neater explanation for this cluster of manifestations than lung cancer. It was a mysterious entity called *sarcoidosis.*

Sarcoidosis is what is known as a *granulomatous* disease, which means that its hallmark is the formation of granulomas. These tumorlike masses are composed largely of two types of immune-system cells—*macrophages* and *lymphocytes*—and fibroblasts, the connective-tissue cells that synthesize collagen. The formation of granulomas represents the body's attempt at repelling an attack. In tuberculosis, a granulomatous disease, the body is mounting a defense against invasion by a particular type of bacteria. In sarcoidosis, the inciting factor is unknown. Just as a disease called *scleroderma* can be thought of as the scarring process gone wild, sarcoidosis is the inflammatory phase of the immune response run amok. Sarcoidosis can attack almost any organ. The lungs and skin are most commonly affected, but tumors and lesions can also appear on the liver, eyes, central nervous system tissue, and bone. People with sarcoidosis often lose a lot of calcium in their urine and frequently develop kidney stones as a result. Ingrid had all the hallmarks of classic sarcoidosis and really none of those of lung cancer. The prognosis for patients with sarcoidosis is a lot better than for patients with metastatic lung cancer. In and of itself, it is rarely fatal.

The cause of sarcoidosis is still unknown. It has been blamed on infections, exposure to specific allergic triggers, hormonal imbalances, or an autoimmune process similar to those believed to cause rheumatoid arthritis or lupus. Some evidence suggests sarcoidosis may be partly genetic, since it occasionally runs in families. Many cases of familial sarcoidosis occur in West Indians, and, in the United States, it is ten times more common in blacks than in whites. Fair-haired Nordics and red-haired Celts also fall prey to it. Sarcoidosis is slightly more common in women, and it usually first becomes apparent between the ages of twenty and forty.

Ingrid's skin lesion, as I remembered it, made me think of *lupus pernio,* or purple lupus, which again fit the whole picture I was developing. Sarcoidosis patients with this type of skin sign seem to have a slightly different variant of the overall disease. I needed to check some references, but as I remembered it, lupus pernio often appeared in conjunction with sarcoidosis that involved the kidneys, upper respiratory tract, and eyes. If I was right, Ingrid was a textbook case.

My heart was pounding with excitement. It all fit so well! If Ingrid had sarcoidosis it would probably be chronic, but it was treatable. We could take care of her.

Making sure the monitors from the babies' rooms were turned on loud so I could hear them, I went across the driveway to the library, where Arthur was furiously scribbling notes. Seeing the intent look on his face, I was hesitant to interrupt him. He put his hand up to indicate that I shouldn't say anything, so I waited in the doorway for a few minutes until he looked up.

"Everything okay?"

"I haven't been able to sleep, because I've been thinking so much about Ingrid. The other day at lunch, just serendipitously, I happened to notice something on her arm. It was a small violaceous plaque. Nothing remarkable, until I remembered she had

had kidney stones—which was mentioned in the report we got from that doctor. . . ."

"You're right," Arthur interrupted. "All of those plus her Swedish ancestry suggest sarcoidosis. That would certainly be a relief. We'll call her tomorrow."

"I know it's late, but I want to call her now. I know she's still at her friend's in Delaware through this week, and I don't want her to leave before we see that spot again."

I dialed the number she had given me. Ingrid herself answered. After exchanging greetings and my apologies for calling so late, I quickly plunged in. "Ingrid, the other day I noticed you had a small purple spot behind your left arm, just below the shoulder. Do you know how long you've had it?"

"What spot? I didn't know I had one at all. But if I'm as sick as that doctor says I am, what does one little skin lesion really matter?"

"It might matter a lot, Ingrid. Look, I don't want to raise false hopes, but from the very beginning I felt you had been misdiagnosed. The whole thing just didn't sit right with me, and I was so upset I couldn't stop thinking about it. And just now it all came together, which is why I am calling you in the middle of the night—kidney stones, lung tumors, the skin lesion, and your being from Sweden. There's a disease called sarcoidosis which combines all those signs and symptoms."

Ingrid sighed. "It's almost frightening to have hope."

"It's frightening for me too, but both Dr. Balin and I feel that sarcoidosis is a strong possibility."

"So what do we do next? My appointment with Dr. Bierman is tomorrow afternoon."

"Don't change that, but I want to biopsy your lesion. As you know we always send tissue samples out to a dermatopathology lab for diagnosis, and we'll do that this time too, but you're family. We'll remove the lesion tomorrow and we'll examine it ourselves. Then we'll proceed from there. Can you come in tomorrow morning first thing—say around eight-thirty?"

"Of course I can. I'd be so grateful." Her voice broke, and I too felt like crying.

I was so excited by the possibility of having found an alternate explanation for Ingrid's cluster of signs and symptoms that, for the briefest instant, I wished I didn't have a breakfast date with Allison. The next morning, as soon as my mother arrived to care for the children, I jumped in my car and sped to the office.

Ingrid was already waiting. I biopsied a piece of her lesion and prepared a slide. My first glimpse through the microscope filled me with elation—there it was, for all to see. I rang for Arthur to come downstairs as soon as he could. When Arthur looked through the microscope, a slow smile spread across his face.

"This makes me feel a lot better. The tissue is loaded with multinucleated giant cells." These are abnormal macrophages, a type of immune cell that engulfs and eats invading cells. (The word macrophage literally means "big eater"). Normal cells have only a single-cell nucleus. The very presence of cells with multiple nuclei is abnormal and generally characteristic of granulomatous diseases, like cutaneous tuberculosis, leprosy, and sarcoidosis, but not lung cancer. "I'd be very surprised if the lung symptomatology was anything but granulomatous in nature," Arthur said, looking up from the microscope.

"Ingrid," I called into the waiting room. "Come see. I want you to look."

As Ingrid peered into the microscope, I said, "What you're seeing is exactly what Dr. Balin and I hoped for. We'll send it out to an independent lab for confirmation, but I feel very comfortable with the diagnosis. I think it's important for you to go have your chest x-ray repeated. But go to Dr. Bierman this time. Then we can discuss your treatment."

Ingrid looked up from the microscope, her eyes shining.

"Oh, Dr. Pratt," she said. "What a gift, what a gift."

That afternoon, Ingrid took the other doctor's report and went to see Dr. Bierman. His report, when it came back, said, "Metastatic disease is unlikely. The appearance of the pulmonary nodules is more suggestive of an old chronic inflammatory process—perhaps sarcoid or granulomatous. This is especially likely in view of the skin biopsy and the patient's history of kidney stones."

With the correct diagnosis finally in, I started Ingrid on the corticosteroids she needed to control her disease. We keep a close eye on her, because the type of sarcoidosis she has can affect the eyes and the nasal septum, the tissue that partitions the nose.

After that trauma, we all breathed a collective sigh of relief and returned to our respective work with a renewed appreciation of the power of a solitary skin lesion to expose the presence of a systemic disease.

Michael Ivanoff was "referred" by Arthur's longtime friend Dick Sternberg. Dick sends many patients Arthur's way. One gentleman who came to our office to have his skin checked did so after meeting Dick on an airplane. When the man learned that Dick was a stockbroker, he had asked him for some tips. Dick had turned to him and said, "Look: the best tip I can give you is to go see Dr. Arthur Balin or his wife, Dr. Loretta Pratt. It might save your life." He had then gone on to deliver our platform on the dangers of sun and press our office telephone number into his startled seatmate's hand. Dick himself was among Arthur's earliest "patients." The first time I met him, he explained to me that it had been evident to all by the time Arthur was twelve years old that he was going to be a doctor like his father and uncles. Dick remembered that, as a boy, Arthur used to schedule appointments with his classmates out on the back stairs of the school, where he would perform finger sticks to draw blood and take it home and type it. Eventually Arthur's parents got wind of the young Doctor Balin's "clinic" and put a stop to it. But Arthur's curiosity was irrepressible. That summer he started a lawn-mowing business, and he used his earnings to set up his first laboratory. Lawn-mowing money in hand, he would walk several miles down the road to a store that sold chemicals and laboratory equipment. Like other children in a candy shop or a record store, Arthur would spend hours browsing and choosing chemicals and equipment with which he was stocking what his father later described as an "impressive" home lab. For Arthur, medicine is far more than a profession. It has always been his destiny.

Arthur, who at the time Michael Ivanoff first came was spending his weekdays in Texas doing his training in Mohs micrographic surgery, referred Michael to me, because the intricacy of Michael's schedule rarely permitted him to get to Pennsylvania on weekends from his home in New York City.

Michael was an international lawyer whom Dick knew from

college. The adage "Work hard, play hard" could have been coined for Michael. He worked an eighty-hour week, often flying between New York, Paris, and Japan in a single week. He had a wife in New York and a girlfriend in Paris, and he made close to a million dollars a year. This information was not elicited in response to any questions I had asked him while taking his history. Michael Ivanoff talked nonstop. It was all I could do to get a word in edgewise to ask him what his skin problem was.

"Itching! I itch all over, all the time. I mean really, sometimes I can't get to sleep because my legs are itching and burning so much. Or even worse, I'll be sitting in a meeting with an important client, and I won't be able to refrain from scratching, and once I start, I often can't stop. I just sit there scratching, like a dog with fleas! The funny thing is that I don't have a rash or anything I can see on my skin, except gouges where I've scratched."

He had gone to his family physician, who had tried a couple of fixes like emollients and steroid creams. Then the physician had done something quite unusual: he had referred Michael to a psychiatrist, explaining that idiopathic (meaning "cause unknown") *pruritus,* like idiopathic pain, might respond to antidepressant medication and a brief course of psychotherapy. Although this is true, I found it surprising that a medical doctor would make such a referral so early on in the diagnostic process.

As the Italian dermatologists Stefano Gatti and Ferdinando Serri remark in the preface to their textbook on pruritus, "In general, the dermatologist should hesitate to suggest an idiopathic or psychological cause for itching. Too frequently this diagnosis cloaks our ignorance in the comforting vestments of an explanation and prevents the discovery of the true cause of a patient's problems that results from detailed investigation."

The psychiatrist had started Michael on an antidepressant called doxepin, which also has antihistamine activity and often improves itching. For nearly six months, he saw Michael weekly for psychotherapy sessions in which they discussed Michael's life without reference to his skin symptom, although Michael frequently found himself in a paroxysm of scratching right there in the psychiatrist's office. After a couple of months, when the doxepin still hadn't controlled the maddening itching, the psychiatrist suggested it was perhaps his guilt about having a girlfriend that was causing Michael to somatize. "I've noticed, Michael, that the scratching seems much worse whenever we talk about Liliane. Maybe this is something we should explore. . . ."

It was at this point, Michael explained to me, "just when I was beginning to think this guy was full of it, that Dick and I had lunch. As usual, I started scratching, and Dick suggested—no not suggested, *insisted*—Dick insisted that I see your husband."

Aside from the pruritus, Michael claimed excellent health. He admitted to feeling somewhat tired a lot of the time, but he attributed this to the long hours in his office and too much time on the Concorde. Michael did say he enjoyed drinking, but except for the "one and a half" martinis he drank each evening, he drank mostly wine. Drinking didn't seem to set off the itching, but one thing he had noticed recently was that he got an immediate pain in the upper right part of his abdomen the moment he tasted his first drink.

"Liliane, like a good Frenchwoman, says it's just *crise de foie,* but at my last checkup, my GP said he couldn't feel my liver, and my blood tests were totally normal. Even my cholesterol is okay."

I, too, wondered whether he might have something going on in his liver. Liver disease doesn't usually cause pain in the area of the liver, but itching is a fairly common symptom of a number of liver diseases. The relationship between itch and jaundice was first noted in the medical literature in A.D. 160 by Aretaeus the Cappodocian. Itching can herald chronic hepatitis, gallbladder stones, and a type of cirrhosis of the liver not related to drinking. But pruritus can be an important diagnostic clue to many other systemic diseases as well. Malignancies, kidney failure, thyroid disease—all may have insatiable itching as a symptom.

Itching is one of the most common complaints for which patients see dermatologists. It's a mysterious phenomenon. Little is understood of its physiology or that of its mirror response, scratching. It is believed that the sensation of itching is transmitted to the central nervous system by nerves that lie in the junction of the dermis and epidermis. Different types of nerve fibers carry the two different types of itch sensations: the sharp, well-localized, usually satiable itch and the diffuse, unpleasant itch that no amount of scratching seems to assuage.

The relationship between itch and pain is also still being debated, with those in one camp believing that itch is merely a vitiated sensation of pain involving the same nerve pathways and the others holding equally tenaciously that pain and itch have nothing in common. Those who support this latter view base their contention on the following observations:

- Both pain and itch can be perceived more or less concurrently in the same spot.
- Opiate painkillers relieve pain but not itch and may even themselves cause insatiable itching.
- The bodily responses to itching and pain are quite different. The former provokes scratching, whereas the latter leads to withdrawal of contact.
- Heating the skin eliminates itch but not pain, just as the removal of an area of epidermis and dermis eliminate itch but not pain. Cooling of the skin relieves pain.

Experts who contend that itching is really a low-grade form of pain base their arguments on the following observations:

- Substances like histamine cause itching when small quantities are injected into the skin and pain when larger amounts are used.
- Individuals who are unable to experience pain also don't experience itching.

Almost equally mysterious in its physiology is scratching, although certainly no mystery surrounds the pleasure to be derived therefrom. The French essayist Montaigne, in his essay "Of Experience," wrote, "Scratching is one of the sweetest gratifications of nature and as ready at hand as any." James I of England made a snootier statement: "None but kings and princes should have the itch, for the sensation of scratching is so delightful."

How scratching relieves itching can still only be speculated upon. It may be that the pain generated by scratching is more bearable than continued itching or that scratching actually destroys nerve endings that are transmitting itching sensations or that it overloads the nerve endings so they cannot simultaneously transmit the itch sensation. The mechanical action of scratching may also rid the skin of parasites and other vectors of itching. Unfortunately, scratching often provides only a quick fix, setting off a spiraling itch-scratch cycle—with itching begetting scratching, which actually enlarges the itchy area, and so on to the point of frenzy.

In my examining room, I carefully read over Michael's health questionnaire as well as the history I had taken. Nothing in his history raised any suspicions. He took no medications and claimed never to have had allergies or hay fever, which might have demonstrated an allergic tendency. His household included no pets, and nothing in his occupation suggested a trigger for the itching. I carefully combed Michael's body for any surface features that might give a clue to the origin of his itching, but I found no rashes, visible lesions, signs of parasites—not even dry skin—that might explain his intense pruritus.

I could clearly see excoriations and scratch marks where he had tried to assuage his itching. Sometimes an astute diagnostician can learn much that is quite specific from the pattern and location of scratch marks. For instance, scratch marks in scabies are typically quite short, which reflects the length of the mites' burrows, while scratch marks in pediculosis, or body lice infestation, tend to be several inches long, in keeping with the greater size of this organism's universe. Patients whose underlying problem is psychological may have deep gouges, or they may have virtually no marks at all, despite dramatic complaints of constant, insatiable itching.

"Is there any time of day when you itch more?" I queried, although he had already told me his paroxysms of itching were unpredictable.

"As I said, it can strike at any time, even at extremely inopportune moments during my workday, but I suppose it does happen more at night—which isn't any treat either."

At this point, Michael presented a clue that really spoke to me: "My sleep is suffering these days," he said. "I'm jet-lagged all the time, so I have insomnia, and if I'm not scratching, I'm sweating. I mean, sometimes I wake up and the sheets are absolutely drenched. The worst is when I wake up itching *and* sweating. My wife is ready to move me into the guest room."

Now things began to make sense, although a disturbing picture was emerging. Night sweats tend to be harbingers of fairly serious diseases: AIDS, TB, cancers. In my mind, the confluence of itching and night sweats weighted my diagnosis more toward a malignancy of the lymphatic system, like non-Hodgkin's lymphoma or Hodgkin's disease. Looking back over his chart, I noted again what he had said about having pain almost immediately after a drink. Somewhere in the back of my mind, I knew this was an idiosyncratic symptom of either some type of leukemia or lymphatic cancer. I made a note to look it up later.

Although my initial exploration of his body had concentrated on surface lesions, I palpated the lymph nodes of his groin, neck, and underarms for any swelling, which would be a typical sign of lymphoma, but I felt nothing. When I had finished my examination, I said, "I don't see anything on your skin that I feel can account for your itching, particularly not itching of such intensity and duration as yours. I think the next step is to do some blood tests, which will give me more information to go on. I want you also to have a chest x-ray and a skin test for TB."

"Why? Do you think I have some kind of real problem? I mean, itching's a drag, but it's not *that* big a deal. Why would you want a chest x-ray? I stopped smoking twelve years ago. No one in my family's had cancer."

"Michael, I don't see any obvious explanation for your itching, so I need to look below the skin. In order to treat you, I have to find the correct diagnosis."

"All right," he said, holding out his arm. "Let's get on with it."

As I drew the blood from a vein in his arm, he regarded the opposite wall and said in a small voice, "You don't think I have AIDS or anything, do you? I just saw that movie *Philadelphia,* and it really scared me. Not that I'm gay or a drug user or anything."

"Have you ever been tested for HIV?"

"No," he said warily. "I'm not sure I really want to be, either."

"It's your call, but I would recommend having a test, since you mentioned having multiple sexual partners."

"All right, all right," he said. "Do whatever you need to do."

When Michael's tests came back, he was negative for HIV, his skin test was negative for TB, and his chest x-rays showed no shadows or calcifications that could have been tumors. What did show was an elevated white blood cell count with some atypical lymphocytes, a type of white blood cell that is an important part of the body's immune surveillance against cancers and foreign proteins. Michael was also borderline anemic.

When Michael was finally able to return my phone call, it was from a hotel room in Kyoto. I told him about his test results.

"Uh-oh, that sounds bad," Michael said, audibly deflated. "Although at least it's not AIDS. That merits an extra martini." Then he cut the wisecracking tone and said, "What do I do next, Dr. Pratt?"

"I would like to consult with your internist about doing some further tests," I said. "It may be more convenient for you to have them done in New York, or I can refer you to a doctor down here. Then, depending upon the outcome of the tests, we'll see if you need to come back to me or whether you should be treated by another physician."

"Dr. Pratt?" he spoke quietly now. "It's cancer, isn't it? You know, don't you? Please tell me your gut feeling."

"My gut feeling is that you may have some type of blood or lymphatic system cancer, but I can't be sure without more tests."

He gave me permission to consult his internist, who decided to refer him to the cancer hospital, Memorial–Sloan Kettering, for further tests.

As it turned out, Michael's itching could very well have saved his life, for in his case, it was the earliest symptom of Hodgkin's disease, a cancer of the lymphatic system. This type of lymphoma is usually curable, particularly when caught early.

A few weeks after I received the report from Michael's internist, which confirmed the diagnosis of Hodgkin's disease, I received a note from Michael. Ever peripatetic, he had faxed it from a hotel room in London. "Dr. Pratt," it said, "I have you to thank. All those other doctors tried, but you got there first. I have every hope of being cured largely because you were on your toes and wasted no time. Thanks."

As of this writing, Michael's cancer has been in remission for five years. He comes in for an annual skin exam and still brings a smile to my face with his outrageous tales of the high life.

In the case of Pilar Ortega, an atypical skin sign was the only clue to what has become a fairly rare diagnosis in the United States. I saw Pilar in the clinic when I was a resident at New York Hospital. Pilar, who was from Colombia, spoke virtually no English, so she had brought her fifteen-year-old American-born nephew, Eduardo, to translate.

"She's here because her ear is hurting her," the nephew explained, "and it keeps getting bigger and bigger."

I gently pulled back the long hair with which Pilar had covered her ear. The ear was a startling sight. The entire pinna, the gristly part above the earlobe, was swollen to three or four times its normal size and was studded with warty excrescences. It appeared at first glance to be some sort of tumor or inflammatory condition, but I had no idea what.

Pilar was thirty-eight years old. She said she had always been healthy until the problem began to develop on her ear.

"I will need to do a biopsy," I said to them. "I will need to take a small piece of the growth on her ear and send it to the laboratory. Tell her not to worry. I'll make her ear numb so it won't hurt." The nephew relayed my words in their rapid, staccato tongue, and Pilar nodded in assent.

The first step in diagnosing a skin lesion is to take a thorough history and then examine the skin. If the diagnosis is not evident, the next step is to obtain a skin biopsy, which is stained to make certain structures and organisms visible by microscope. The biopsy usually helps determine what category of lesion we are seeing—for instance, whether it is a tumor, infection, or inflammation.

The dermatopathology report stated that the growth was a caseating granuloma—again, a description but not a diagnosis. This description suggested a number of diagnoses—most classically, tuberculosis. However, Pilar's complaint was so unusual that I suspected another explanation. The next step was to send some of the tissue sample to be cultured, meaning that the sample is put in a culture medium to feed and encourage the growth of any bacteria present, to the point where their numbers are high enough to be detectable. Different growth media can be used, with many microorganisms being rather finicky about exactly which type of food they prefer. It requires about fifteen weeks and a special medium to culture the bacteria that cause tuberculosis from a sample of sputum or tissue. Then a special stain is used to preferentially color the bacteria that cause TB. The stain renders them pinkish-red; hence the pathologists' name for them: "red snappers." Because pathologists must work from such a small piece of tissue, specimens may contain few organisms, and those present may be quite elusive.

At the same time I sent the culture down to the lab, I decided more information might be gleaned from Pilar herself. With her nephew's help, I said to her, "We still aren't certain what is causing the growth on your ear, and we need your help. Have you ever had tuberculosis, or have you ever been exposed to it?"

At this point, Pilar's face lost the pleasant but slightly uncomprehending smile she had been maintaining, and a shadow of fear passed across it. She said something emphatic to her translator.

"My aunt says she is not sick in that way."

"Ask her if she has ever been around anyone who has been sick with tuberculosis."

Still she shook her head no. But something about the vehemence of her denial aroused my suspicions. In countries where TB is still rampant, to be infected with it is often a source of shame, because it is associated with poverty, overcrowding, and poor sanitation. It occurred to me also that Pilar was probably worried we might hospitalize her or perhaps report her to Immigration.

"Tell her it's not a problem, but if she has been exposed, we need to know so we can treat her. Tell her there are drugs that treat the disease if she does have it."

The two conversed for a moment. "She still says she isn't sick. She once took care of an old woman who might have had it, because she coughed all the time and then she died, but she says she has never been sick like that."

Tuberculosis—the dramatic "consumption" of nineteenth-century novels—while largely eradicated in most groups in the United States at that time, the mid-1980s, was still widespread in other parts of the world. In countries where milk is not routinely pasteurized, TB can be transmitted by infected cows. Even more common is airborne transmission. The bacteria can float in room air for several hours after an infected person has departed, infecting passersby without their even knowing they were exposed.

While most people think of TB as a disease of the lungs—and indeed, it most often is—TB can also infect virtually any other organ, including bone.

In countries where TB is still a problem, large segments of the population are vaccinated against it with *bacille Calmette-Guerin* (BCG), a vaccine prepared from the bacterium that causes tuberculosis in cows, *Mycobacterium bovis.* To submit a patient who has been given this vaccine to the standard skin test can cause a violently positive response, with inflammation and eventual tissue death at the test site as the patient's antibodies battle it out with the bacterial antigens, using the skin as a battlefield. Since many South American countries had vaccination programs in those days, I needed to know whether Pilar had been vaccinated before I considered a skin test. But when I asked, with Eduardo's help, she said she had had so many shots, she didn't really know. I decided little conclusive information was to be gained by attempting a skin test. If she had had the vaccine, she would have a positive skin test, although it could be a false positive, indistinguishable from a true positive. In any case, a skin test would only demonstrate whether or not she had ever been exposed to TB and not whether she presently had an active infection. We needed the results of the culture to really tell if we were seeing a case of extrapulmonary TB.

At last, the culture results were available. To my great interest, the culture was negative: no growth. At this point, the pathologist at Cornell who had been working on the case felt we needed some help. We decided to obtain some more skin samples and run another in-house culture, while at the same time we sent slides and tissue specimens to the Armed Forces Institute of Pathology, in Washington. The AFIP has one of the most extensive and authoritative pathology collections in the United States. It's considered the gold standard for diagnosis.

We then settled in to wait another long fifteen weeks while the cultures were growing. Pilar's skin lesion continued to spread slowly up to her scalp. I sent her for chest x-rays to see whether we might find some sign of active disease there, but there were no nodules, no fluid infiltrates, and no scars.

TB is a stealthy disease, a characteristic that made it an excellent candidate to become epidemic. As is also true of syphilis,

ninety percent or more of initial TB infections are virtually asymptomatic and go unrecognized. There may be a sense of not feeling
entirely well or coldlike signs and symptoms, but not much more,
to mark the entry of *Mycobacterium tuberculosis* into the human
body. Once established, TB may lie dormant for years and flare up
at some later point. Most of the cases of TB we were seeing in
adults in the mid-1980s were such recrudescent infections. Nowadays, a resurgence of TB is concurrent with the AIDS epidemic,
and many more adults are acquiring primary infections. At this
writing, TB is still on the rise, particularly in the elderly, the poor,
and the immunocompromised, three groups with much overlap
amongst themselves. This present epidemic is particularly worrisome, because the TB bacterium has developed resistance to some
of the first-choice drugs capable of treating it. Like so many bacteria in the fifty years since antibiotics were first introduced, TB has
managed to learn how to inactivate or block antibiotics faster than
new drugs are being developed. But back in 1985, we weren't
thinking about any of this with regard to TB. TB was still in check,
and we rarely saw it. In fact, in those days, many medical students
had never seen a single case of it.

Pilar, meanwhile, was quite understandably becoming worried
and impatient. By now it had been over six months since her first
visit, and we still couldn't even tell her what was wrong and what
we could do to stop the spread of the lesion. It was clear to all of
us that it *was* spreading, but all we could do was wait and reassure
her until we had a definite diagnosis. Certainly she had no other
signs or symptoms of TB, and until we had identified a microor-
ganism and determined its drug sensitivity, to try to treat it on
suspicion of TB would have been like skeet shooting in the dark.

I did my best to reassure Pilar through a Spanish-speaking
nurse that we were actively seeking the answer and needed her to
bear with us a few more weeks while the cultures grew.

"It's getting so hard to hide it," was all Pilar said.

After Pilar's appointment that afternoon, I was passing by the
patients' cafeteria on my way to the medical library. Looking in, I
saw Pilar and Eduardo. They were eating at a table in the corner.
Pilar, who had taken to wearing a hat pulled down below her ears,
was sitting next to the wall. There was something so bleak and sad
in the picture that I hurried on, knowing there was nothing I could

say, fervently wishing the tests would come back and that, this time, they would tell us something.

Finally our lab had results, and within a few days the report came from AFIP. The organisms in Pilar's ear were *M. tuberculosis,* the bacillus (or rod-shaped bacterium) that causes human tuberculosis.

"Pilar, we finally have news for you," the nurse and I told her at her next visit. "You have a very unusual type of tuberculosis."

She looked horrified. Before I could even go on, she burst into Spanish with the nurse.

"She is asking whether she is going to die or whether she could have given the disease to other people in her family. They all live together."

"No," I said. "Tell her that we can treat her. I have to run one more test, but it will only take a few days. I have to find out which drugs will work for her." I also conveyed to her that we could test the other family members and treat them as needed. But Pilar burst into tears and continued to wail for several minutes, every so often stopping to take a breath and say something to the nurse.

"She's saying you don't understand. The type of TB in her country kills people. She is afraid you won't be able to cure her. She is asking why you can't just remove her ear, that maybe the disease hasn't spread yet."

I took Pilar's hand in mine until her sobs finally subsided into silent streams of tears that continued to run down her face. "Pilar," I said to her, with both the nurse and Eduardo translating, "I know you have seen people die from this disease. Many people used to die in this country too, but it doesn't happen when people are treated. I promise you we'll be able to treat you and your family if need be. And you will not lose your ear. You will see in a few months that your ear will start to look better. By this time next year, you will never know you had a problem." She looked up at me and burst into tears again. The nurse put her arm around her shoulders and reiterated all I had said.

As soon as the sensitivity testing was completed, I started Pilar on triple antibiotic therapy. Over the course of about a year, during which time she continued to take the three drugs, the large and dramatic lesion slowly disappeared. By the end of her antibiotic therapy, the ear looked exactly like its unaffected mate.

Toward the end of her therapy, when her ear was clearly healing, Pilar turned to me and said in English, "Still I do not understand. Why did this disease come into my skin?" Then she sat back so that I could speak directly with Eduardo.

"Tell her she might have gotten it from the old lady or from someone else who had the disease and didn't know it. The TB might have gotten into her skin through a cut or by kissing someone who was sick."

Pilar had a type of tuberculosis of the skin known as *lupus vulgaris*. While most people are more familiar with the word *lupus* in the setting of the disease *lupus erythematosus*, lupus is actually a descriptive term whose original meaning in medicine was a lesion that looked as though it had been gnawed by wolves, *lupus* being the Latin for wolf. Many skin manifestations described as lupoid, in their end stages, looked very much like something that had been savagely attacked. Some say that the term is used in connection with lupus erythematosus because of the characteristic skin rash spread across the nose and cheekbones. While some call this a butterfly rash, others feel that its shape resembles the mask of a wolf.

Lupus vulgaris is the most common type of cutaneous TB and the most disfiguring. It is chronic and progresses slowly, but incessantly, over decades. Left untreated, it would have been extremely disfiguring. The lesions of lupus vulgaris can ulcerate and destroy large areas of supporting cartilage, so that the nose may be destroyed or the opening of the mouth may become so small and contracted that eating and speech become nearly impossible. One of the most serious and frequent complications of long-term lupus vulgaris is squamous cell carcinoma.

Although Pilar's TB was limited to her skin, most patients with lupus vulgaris have TB in some other organ as well. It used to be thought that lupus vulgaris actually conferred some immunity against TB in other organs and that it was a good sign. However, that thinking was not borne out by experience. In many cases, lupus vulgaris may actually mean that TB in some other organ is running a serious course.

Pilar's story often comes to mind as I think about the many patients I can recall whose systemic diseases were revealed only by a skin change. I shudder to think, sometimes, how many patients are receiving unnecessary treatments or are not getting the treatment they really need, just because their doctors are not conversant in the language of skin. Ted Jenks, a patient of Arthur's is a prime example.

Not long after Arthur and I were married, we went to Hawaii for a few days' vacation following a medical meeting in San Francisco. Arthur is a certified scuba diving instructor, though it's a passion he rarely gets the chance to indulge. We had gotten off the plane a couple of hours earlier and had decided to unwind by going for a walk on the beach. I remember Arthur was still wearing the suit he had worn on the plane, and I was wearing a long skirt, with my shirt sleeves rolled down and a big hat. Although clothing does not substitute for sunblock, it does add some ultraviolet protection with its SPF of about 7. People in bathing suits walking in the surf and others roasting themselves on towels stared at us as we made our way along the beach. To them, I supposed, we looked rather outlandish—like the occasional Amish farmers we see near our home in Pennsylvania or the veiled women in Muslim countries. I remembered a time when I, too, would have been among them on a beach blanket of my own with a pile of medical school textbooks and a little tube of SPF 4 to keep my face from burning.

We were just walking next to a grove of low tropical bushes when we heard a voice proclaim, "Those two look like a couple of dermatologists on vacation." And out from the deepest shade ambled Ted Jenks, a patient of Arthur's who had a condominium nearby. Ted himself was wearing a big straw hat and long sleeves, and he transferred a large bottle of SPF 30 sunblock into his left hand to greet us.

Ted had been a patient of Arthur's for many years. He had been referred to Arthur as a last resort after he had made the rounds of nearly a dozen physicians of all specialties. To Arthur's eye, Ted Jenks's skin was fairly screaming the diagnosis, but its communications had been ignored or misunderstood for many years.

The first sign of Ted's illness had been a reddish lesion in the shape of an inverted V on his back. "It just kind of popped out of my skin one day. It was my wife who noticed it."

Ted, who was an electrical engineer for a large corporation outside Baltimore, went to see his company's doctor. "He didn't seem very worried," he told Arthur. "In fact, I got the impression he thought I was kind of a crybaby for coming in to have it looked at in the first place, but my wife was worried it might be some kind of cancer, because I spent a lot of time in the sun." The employer's physician had reassured Ted that what he had did not resemble a skin cancer or anything dangerous. He gave Ted some cortisone cream and told him to get some sun and air on his back. That was in early 1977, when Ted was in his mid-forties. Over the course of the year the mark faded, and everyone forgot about it—until a year later, when it reappeared. This time, the inverted V was darker and more purple, and a few other similar spots seemed to be developing on his chest and back. Again he was sent to the company doctor. This time, Ted was given barrages of tests. "I had bone marrow tests, lymphangiograms, biopsies, every blood test in the book, and they still had no idea what was the matter with me. The best they could come up with was some kind of cancer. So I was referred to some cancer specialists in Baltimore. They redid a lot of the same tests, and they, too, were more or less stumped. Eventually, they did another skin biopsy and decided it was lymphoma of the skin." The oncologists recommended a course of radiation therapy, but Ted declined, insisting on another opinion first, because he felt just fine. "There was no way I was going to let them just start zapping me with radiation when they didn't even have a diagnosis that everyone agreed on. As far as I was concerned, I just had some kind of skin rash. I was beginning to wish I hadn't even opened the whole can of worms," he said with a laugh. He was referred to a physician in Philadelphia for another opinion. Unfortunately, by the time Ted saw her, his lesion had again begun to recede. The doctor and he decided to keep an eye on it but do nothing. Within a few months of no treatment, nothing much was left on Ted's skin with which to make a diagnosis. He decided to stay away from doctors.

The lesion remained more or less invisible for several years. But when it returned after a vacation in Hawaii, it did so with a vengeance, accompanied by smaller lesions all over his face and back. This time, when Ted was sent to the company doctor, the doctor referred him to a new young dermatologist in town named Arthur

Balin. Since Arthur's father and uncles had been physicians in Chester for many years, the Balin name was familiar to local physicians.

Arthur is board certified in six specialties—internal medicine, dermatology, dermatopathology, geriatric medicine, Mohs micrographic surgery and cutaneous oncology, and dermatologic cosmetic surgery. He also holds a Ph.D. in biochemistry. He is one of very few doctors in this country to be certified in so many specialties, and this combination gives him a unique perspective. As soon as he laid eyes on Ted Jenks and heard his story, he had a strong suspicion that Ted had some form of lupus erythematosus. The tip-off was the fact that the characteristic marks on his skin were worsened by sun exposure. Furthermore, the appearance of the scaly reddish and purple plaques on Ted's back, ears, and chest, in conjunction with this history, fairly screamed the diagnosis. Although some form of lupus was at the top of Arthur's list and he decided to pursue this diagnosis first, it was always possible that Ted did have cutaneous lymphoma. Psoriasis was also a consideration, since several of Ted's family members had it.

"Ted, I know you're probably getting pretty tired of blood tests and people taking pieces of your skin," Arthur said, "but I think we'll be able to get a firm diagnosis this time."

"What's your thought?" he asked.

"I'm most suspicious of some type of lupus, but I don't want to commit myself to that until we get the test results. You certainly have some of the classic signs."

"What *is* lupus, Dr. Balin? It's one of those words you hear around and don't pay any attention to until it has something to do with you."

Arthur explained to him that lupus erythematosus is a condition in which a person makes antibodies against his own DNA—the genetic information we carry in the nucleus of every cell. These inappropriate antibodies are known as anti-DNA and antinuclear antibodies. Lupus, like rheumatoid arthritis, is what is known as an autoimmune disease, meaning that the patient's own immune system ceases to recognize some cells or parts of cells as native and, instead, mounts the sort of attack it would when repelling a foreign protein. As with rheumatoid arthritis, the disease process has been identified, but what actually makes the immune system attack the tissues it is supposed to be protecting remains a mystery. Other diseases, however, may provide a clue. One of these is rheumatic fever, an inflammatory disease that can occur as a delayed sequel to strep infection of the throat. Its typical symptoms include arthritis in multiple joints, fever, and inflammation of the heart. It has now been shown that portions of certain streptococci bacteria bear an immunologic resemblance to portions of human cells. The successful immune defense mounted to repel these bacterial invaders can turn out to be a Pyrrhic victory when, after the strep organisms in the body have been killed, the antibodies produced for that effort turn against their host and destroy the heart valves. While this model may not serve to explain the autoimmune process that takes place in lupus, it is one of the first instances in which the mystery of the seemingly mutinous immune system has been explained.

"Doctor, if I do turn out to have lupus, then what's my future?"

"There are two types of lupus, Ted. One is called discoid lupus, and it affects only the skin. The other is called systemic lupus, and it can attack not only the skin but also any of the internal organs. First, I will determine from the biopsies I just took whether or not you have either type of lupus. If lupus is confirmed, I will need to biopsy a bit of uninvolved skin in order to tell you which type you have. If you have discoid lupus, there won't be any of the typical antibodies in your uninvolved skin, only in the lesions themselves."

"I hope you don't mind my asking all these questions, but I'm curious. Why did you take a blood test too, if what you need to know is in my skin?"

"The blood tests will give me additional useful information. For instance, very often in discoid lupus there are no antinuclear antibodies circulating in the blood. Blood tests also give a lot of nonspecific information that can help me determine what's going on, especially if it turns out that you don't have lupus. I ordered a complete blood count with a differential. The complete blood count tells me how many red and white blood cells and platelets you have. The differential tells about the levels and ratios of various types of white blood cells. It can tell me whether you have an active infection. It may also tell me whether you have some problem with your white blood cells or your immune system. The erythrocyte sedimentation rate test is nonspecific, but it, too, tells me whether there is an inflammatory reaction. I also ordered a biochemical profile, which can help point out specific abnormalities in organ function if you have abnormal levels of certain wastes or by-products or if your levels of various minerals are off. The biochemical profile gives us a kind of map, so that we know to look in some particular organ."

"That's interesting. You know, in all the time people have been taking blood out of my body for testing, I've never asked, because I never thought anyone would bother to give me an answer I could understand. That's a compliment, by the way," he said with a grin.

Arthur thanked him and told him he would be in touch as soon as he had some results.

A week later, he had some answers. In their microscopic appearance, the biopsies taken from the lesions were classically indicative of lupus. That was partially reassuring, but any systemic involvement still had to be ascertained. Arthur brought Mr. Jenks back in for another biopsy. This time, he removed one sample from one of the lesions and another from normal skin on the inside of Ted's upper arm.

"At this point, Ted, we know that you have some type of lupus," Arthur told him, "so I'm going to give you some steroid cream to help heal the lesions themselves. I'll have an exact diagnosis for you after I have the results of the immunofluoresence test."

The immunofluoresence test would reveal whether or not there were immune deposits along the base of the epidermis. If they were found to be present in the normal skin from Ted Jenks's arm, a diagnosis of systemic lupus would be clear. If not, it could safely be said that Mr. Jenks had a condition confined to his skin.

A few days later, Arthur got word that no antibodies had been found in Ted's normal skin.

While the diagnosis meant Ted wasn't suffering from the life-threatening form of lupus, discoid lupus itself is a serious diagnosis. It can be extremely disfiguring, particularly if left untreated. Lesions that begin as scattered red plaques can later coalesce into large areas of ulceration that eventually heal, often with severe scarring. Discoid lupus frequently attacks the inside of the mouth and the lips as well as the conjunctiva, the membrane that lines the eyes. It can also extend into the scalp and cause irreversible hair loss.

"As I had hoped, Ted, the tests show that you have the form of lupus limited to the skin. Since the steroid cream has been helping clear the lesions, I want you to keep using it on any active areas. But I also want to start you on an oral medication that will help control your disease. It's a drug called Plaquenil, and although it was developed to treat malaria, it's one of the better treatments available for lupus as well. Before you start, I would like you to see an ophthalmologist for an examination, just to be certain that your eyes are normal, because this drug can cause eye problems. You'll also need to have your eyes rechecked every three months while you're on the medication."

Ted Jenks sat back in his chair, his arms folded behind his head. "Well, well, well," he said. "You know, I can't help but wonder why all those other doctors couldn't figure this one out. Don't you people all go to the same medical schools? What if I *had* gone along and let those cancer doctors do radiation treatment on those first spots? They could have *given* me cancer instead of cured it!"

Arthur, who is always very diplomatic, said nothing.

"Aside from the medications, the other important thing for you to remember is to protect yourself from the sun. We don't understand why it is yet, but for some reason, sunlight can exacerbate this disease and cause flare-ups."

"That's not exactly what I wanted to hear, Dr. Balin. My wife and I just got a condo in Hawaii. We're planning to spend at least a month out there every winter. I've been looking forward to some warm winters for years. So has my wife. I can't disappoint her now."

"I'm not saying you have to change anything about your lifestyle except what you do in the sun. You can protect yourself with a high-SPF sunblock, sunglasses, a hat, and clothing."

And that was how it came to be that we encountered Ted Jenks on that beach in Hawaii, the only other person out there as covered up as we were.

I have chosen to tell the stories of these three patients because they always remind me that the skin is, above all, an organ of communication. As dermatologists, we are fluent in the language of skin. And it is perhaps the most expressive organ of the body. One ignores its communications at one's peril.

Turtle Woman: A Story of Collagen Gone Awry

⟨◎⟩

"As Gregor Samsa awoke one morning from a troubled dream, he found himself changed in his bed. . . . He lay on his back which was as hard as armor plate, and raising his head a little, he could see the arch of his great brown belly, divided by bowed corrugations."

FRANZ KAFKA,
THE METAMORPHOSIS

I once saw a patient who, in not quite as short a time as Gregor Samsa, underwent a startling and terrifying metamorphosis of her own. Each time I recall her, I think of the peculiar predicament we face as physicians when we encounter a rare and fascinating medical problem and, just for a moment, the scientist in us overwhelms the healer. But it is the healer who quickly takes over. Our goal as scientists and researchers is to understand all we can about the natural history of the skin and its disorders. In this capacity, our role is to observe. But as doctors, our goal—indeed, our oath—is to heal our patients as quickly as we can. As dermatologists, we are ever mindful of our patients' appearance and their self-image. To forget the human need to look normal would be to neglect a large part of our job. We see people at their most vulnerable. They come telling us, "I hurt" or "I am frightened, because my skin is changing and I no longer recognize myself."

Elaine Howard was a high school history teacher in her late

· 53 ·

fifties. Until the point at which I met her, she had enjoyed lifelong good health. Her husband had died suddenly five years earlier, but she had carried on, grateful that she was healthy and capable of sustaining herself and her two teenage sons. Then, deep within her skin, something quietly went awry. Slowly, and then with gathering speed, Elaine found herself trapped inside a body that became more gruesome, more alien, by the day.

She arrived in my office clearly distraught. For two years, she said, she had had two small patches of shiny skin, one on her abdomen and the other under her breast. When she first noticed them, she consulted her family physician, who saw nothing to worry about. Elaine accepted his reassurance, and he appeared to have been correct. The patches stayed exactly the same, neither changing nor bothering her for nearly two years. Eventually she forgot about them. But then, quite suddenly, Elaine's metamorphosis began.

"I guess the first change I noticed was the roughness of my skin," she told me at our first meeting. "Still, I didn't think too much about it. My doctor suggested I use a lotion with lactic acid in it to soften up my skin, and even though it didn't really help, I wasn't particularly worried. At that point, it was just like a bad case of very dry skin, which was a little unusual to have happen in the summer, but I was busy getting ready for the opening of school, and I didn't really focus on it too much."

Bit by bit, the patches of shiny skin enlarged. "One morning as I was getting dressed, I noticed more of it on my chest and neck. I didn't do anything about it, because I just didn't have time to get to the doctor and—stupidly, I guess—I still wasn't very worried."

Next, Elaine developed a constellation of small blisters on her arm. This time, she consulted a dermatologist.

"He seemed to be in such a hurry," she said. "So I didn't point out the shiny patches and the rough skin. I didn't think they mattered very much. I couldn't see how they could possibly be connected to the blisters on my arm. At that point, I mainly wanted to get rid of them, because they were quite unattractive and they hurt a lot if I rolled onto my arm while I was sleeping."

The dermatologist diagnosed a staph infection and put Elaine on antibiotics, which cleared up the blisters within a week. "What

I didn't tell him was that my skin also felt tight all over. There wasn't anything peculiar that you could see, but it just felt unusually snug. I didn't really know how to explain it to him, and it actually sounded a little crazy."

"Didn't he ask you to get undressed so that he could examine all your skin?" I asked.

"No, he didn't. But that's my fault, I guess. I only showed him the blisters."

"Elaine, can you describe for me what these patches of skin felt like?" I asked.

"Probably the best way I can describe it is to say that the skin on my arms and legs felt like it was a size too small. It was a bit like wearing clothes that had shrunk in the wash."

Each week it got a little worse, and then it began to get worse very quickly. Elaine said she felt as though the skin over her knees and elbows and shoulders was being stretched to the breaking point. "I felt like someone could scratch me with a knife and I'd pop open," she said. "I could sit in a tub of bath oil all day, but nothing helped."

Within a few months, Elaine's skin became so tight she could barely bend from the waist or lift her arms. The skin on her back was the most affected. Very quickly, it went from being tight and tough to being as hard and thick as leather. Elsewhere on her body, old scars and stretch marks began to be more noticeable. "That's when it hit me—" she said, "—this is *real*. Something is really wrong, and it's beginning to pick up speed. It's becoming torture to go to work in the morning. I can't move very well, and even wearing underwear is almost intolerable—all that elastic digging into me." Her eyes brimmed. "I'm really worried. I don't feel like myself anymore."

The fact that Loretta and I practice in the same building means not only that we get more glimpses of one another throughout the day we would by most any other arrangement, but also that we are able to consult on one another's cases. In this instance, I thought Loretta's calming presence might be helpful to Elaine, and I knew Loretta would be fascinated by Elaine's case. If Elaine was suffering from what I suspected, the speed with which her symptoms were developing made her case unusual.

I rang Loretta's office and found her at her desk going over some biopsy reports on a fifteen-year-old girl she had been worried about.

"Oh good," she said, "I needed to talk to you. The path report on the Simons girl came back positive for mycosis fungoides." (This is a type of skin cancer that occasionally spreads to the internal organs.) "Her involvement is very limited, and I think she'll respond well to topical therapy. The problem is that she has a history of depression and I'm not sure how she's going to react to the news. I want to arrange a family conference to discuss her diagnosis. What do you think?"

"Let's talk about it later when we can sit down together. Right now, there's a very interesting patient in my examining room. Do you have time to come up?"

I ran through possible diagnoses in my mind. Elaine's symptoms were most consistent with those of a group of diseases called scleroderma, in which the skin thickens and hardens. I remembered with sadness the first patient I saw with this condition. She was still vivid in my mind's eye: an elderly woman in a hospital bed surrounded by a group of curious young doctors, myself among them. The disease had hardened the skin around her rib cage so much that she couldn't breathe normally. Her brave, apprehensive face drifted into my mind as Loretta and I went in to examine Elaine.

"Mrs. Howard, this is my wife, Dr. Pratt," I said.

Elaine looked at Loretta's outstretched hand and buried her face in her palms.

"Oh, I feel like such a freak," she said. "I know you have to look at me, but I'm embarrassed to be seen."

Loretta put her hand on Elaine's shoulder. "Relax. You're safe here, Elaine," she said gently.

Both Loretta and I are mindful of the terrible self-consciousness that torments so many of our patients. Throughout history, people with visible skin disease have been shunned and even locked away. The boy or girl afflicted with cystic acne, the otherwise pretty woman with psoriasis who sheds "fish scales" wherever she goes, the man with dandruff on his collar—all are avoided, even mocked, in part because of the deep, self-protective human instinct to stay away from those with unhealthy skin. Loretta and I both believe human touch is an essential component of all healing, but nowhere is it more acutely needed than among our patients, who so often feel themselves to be loathsome and untouchable. We never greet patients without shaking their hands, which, for some of them, is the first forthright touch they have received in a long time.

Elaine's arms and trunk appeared hard and shiny, as if someone had spilled wax on her, but when we looked at her back, we were astounded. The skin there resembled a turtle's carapace more than it did anything human. It was hard and leathery and unyielding.

"Elaine," I said, "we need to get a better idea of what's going on. I want to take a couple of skin biopsies from different locations, and I would like to draw some blood for testing."

Elaine's face, which had been merely apprehensive, flooded with panic.

"*Biopsy?* You don't think I have cancer, do you?"

"No, I don't think you have cancer. There are a couple of diseases that can cause the skin to harden the way yours has. I can't tell you much more until we get your test results back. It will only take a couple of days, and I'll call you as soon as I have them."

"Isn't there anything you can do for me *today?*" Elaine implored. "I mean, even just some kind of cream that would at least make my skin *feel* better?"

One of the most difficult aspects of being a doctor is to adhere to the correct diagnostic procedure when you desperately want to make a person feel better as quickly as you can. To deviate from the diagnostic methods so strongly inculcated in medical school would ultimately be a disservice to the patient, because sometimes medical problems really aren't what they seem to be. This was one of those cases in which I wished I could just sidestep the biopsy and waiting for test results and get on with helping Elaine, but without a diagnosis, I could start her on incorrect treatment, which could further obfuscate the real problem. Clearly, none of the usual skin-softening agents was going to work. This wasn't a simple case of dry skin. Elaine's skin changes were taking place far below the surface.

I took four biopsies from different locations, three from Elaine's chest and one from her back. These four samples represented four different stages of the disease, the skin on her back being the hardest and most advanced. I also ordered a complete blood screen, some specific antibody tests, and one or two other blood tests that might help me confirm my suspicions or rule out other possibilities.

We said good-bye to Elaine and made an appointment for the end of the week, when I would have her dermatopathology report and blood work in hand.

In the car on the way home that night, Loretta turned to me and said, "That poor Mrs. Howard. I keep thinking about her. She must be so frightened. I've seen patients with scleroderma before, but I've never seen anything like the skin on her back."

"My gut feeling is that she does have some type of scleroderma, but there are certainly other possibilities."

Scleroderma is a descriptive term that means "thickening of the skin." Earlier names for hardened skin included *pachydermatous disease* and *elephantiasis scleroderma.* The first published account of a patient with this disease dates from 1752, when a seventeen-year-old girl was admitted to the Royal Hospital in Naples. The skin on her body was hard and tight, and it had even affected her face to the point where she could barely open her mouth or bend her neck. Her physician at the time, a Dr. Curzio, had little at his disposal besides warm milk, vapor baths, small doses of mercury, and bloodletting. After eleven months of these "treatments," her skin was once again soft and pliable. Although Dr. Curzio must have congratulated himself on her cure, we now know that many cases of scleroderma disappear on their own after months or even years.

The thickening skin of scleroderma is caused by greatly stepped-up collagen formation. An added complication is that this may occur not just in the skin but in other organs as well. It is rather like a generalized scarring that occurs in response to no apparent trauma. Scleroderma actually comprises a cluster of diseases: a systemic form, which can be progressive and life-threatening and involve vital organs like the kidneys, heart and lungs, and a localized form, known as morphea.

Morphea itself has three variants. *Linear scleroderma,* the most common of the three, creates bandlike patterns on the skin. When it involves the face, it frequently describes a pale swath that looks like the wound left by a sword. Hence its French name, *en coup de sabre.* Because of the extensiveness of Elaine's skin lesions, if she did indeed have one of the sclerodermas, it was likely she had generalized morphea, the rarest of the three. Because of its extreme rarity, I had seen only three or four cases of it during my twenty years of practice.

"What I'm really worried about," I said, as I turned off the highway and onto the wooded back road where we live, "is the possibility of systemic involvement if she does have scleroderma. She mentioned she's had chronic constipation for the first time in her life over the past year, but she claims she has no trouble swallowing or breathing. I'll be more comfortable when we get the lab work back, but even if it rules out systemic involvement, I still want to send her for esophageal motility and lung function tests just to be certain."

People with the systemic form of scleroderma almost always develop digestive difficulties, because the same process that causes the hardening and thickening of the skin can occur throughout the length of the gastrointestinal tract. The opening of the mouth may become smaller, due to stiffening of the facial skin. When this happens, eating and even smiling may become difficult. Swallowing is frequently impaired, and many patients suffer from chronic heartburn, constipation, and abdominal pain, because the alimentary canal functions more slowly, allowing its contents to pool and become impacted. The heart, lungs, and kidneys can also develop fibrous scar tissue, which affect their function to varying degrees, depending upon the location and extent of the damage. At its worst, this disease gradually suffocates people within rigid, armored bodies, slowly hardening from the outside in. We can do little for them aside from managing their symptoms as best we are able.

"Scleroderma or morphea seems most likely, but what else do you think she could have?"

Actually, several diseases could make a person's skin harden. Years ago, a cluster of cases of *eosinophilia-myalgia syndrome* had developed after people took contaminated batches of the amino acid L-tryptophan, but this supplement had been withdrawn several years before Elaine's symptoms began, and Elaine had denied taking any vitamins at all. There was *scleredema of Buschke,* which had dermal symptoms similar to Elaine's, but this condition usually came on more quickly and resolved more quickly. Also, symptoms were often preceded by a flulike syndrome. Another possibility was *eosinophilic fasciitis,* which can resemble scleroderma, except that it usually has a sudden, often painful, onset and affects the deeper layers of skin and muscle. Occasionally, patients with lupus, diabetes, and other autoimmune diseases—in which the body's immune system unaccountably turns on itself—will develop hard, tight skin. But Elaine had no personal or family history of rheumatoid arthritis or any of the autoimmune diseases. In fact, she told me, except for mild hypertension, which was controlled with a beta blocker, she had always been "ridiculously healthy" and had rarely missed even a day of work.

"Another reason I think she has localized scleroderma, rather than the systemic type, is that she doesn't have Raynaud's phenomenon." Raynaud's phenomenon is common, particularly in women, and is due to spasms in the arterioles, the smallest blood vessels of the arterial system, which carry oxygenated blood from the heart to all the tissues of the body. Attacks may be brought on by emotional upsets as well as by exposure to cold. When attacks occur, the skin of the fingers, toes, and sometimes the tip of the nose goes through a series of color changes corresponding to alterations in the circulation. First, the skin blanches as blood vessel spasms reduce the blood flow to the skin. It then turns blue, because of oxygen starvation, and finally it flushes, as the blood vessel spasms subside and circulation is restored to the affected skin. Raynaud's phenomenon is not serious in and of itself, but it often accompanies serious diseases and needs to be investigated. Patients with systemic scleroderma almost always have Raynaud's phenomenon, while those with the localized form of the disease rarely do.

"Did you order a Lyme disease test?" Loretta asked.

"I did, but I doubt it will come back positive. Elaine's a real city person. When I asked her, she couldn't even remember the last time she had been to the country."

Although the subject of Lyme disease in general is mired in controversy, a few reports in the medical literature have suggested that the tick-borne bacterium *Borrelia burgdorferi* may be involved in morphea. Several studies showed that patients with morphea had antibodies to *B. burgdorferi,* and one study actually revealed Lyme bacteria in the skin lesions of patients with morphea. But most of the time, morphea arises more mysteriously and can't be attributed to any particular infectious agent. Nevertheless, I would have been remiss if I hadn't checked Elaine Howard for Lyme disease.

Elaine's blood work, when it came back, revealed none of the antibodies that might indicate systemic disease. I was also able to rule out lupus, diabetes, Lyme disease, and a form of scleroderma known as CREST, which has many of the same symptoms as systemic scleroderma but progresses more slowly.

Her biopsy report, which came a couple of days later, agreed with the blood work. When I examined the slides prepared from the biopsy material, I could see that the outer layer of Elaine's skin, the epidermis, was quite normal in appearance, but the entire dermis was thickened and contained abnormal numbers of collagen fibers.

Collagen is a protein found throughout the bodies of all mammals. When you look at a piece of leather, what you are actually seeing is the collagen from the animal's dermis. The word *collagen* is derived from the Greek word *kolla,* or glue, which collagen fibers yield when boiled. More than just glue, living collagen is a sort of physiologic mortar that provides the framework for all our tissues, from skin to bone. Without it, we would simply fall apart.

Collagen is familiar to most people as a cosmetic component. Many expensive skin creams boast of their collagen content, but in fact there is no way that collagen spread on the skin can possibly be absorbed. Instead, it is often injected directly into the skin around the mouth and upper lip to plump out wrinkles.

Scleroderma, morphea, and many other autoimmune diseases involve collagen and connective tissues throughout the body. Their symptoms and individual names depend upon the location of the affected tissues, but they are classified as collagen vascular diseases. For example, in rheumatoid arthritis, the immune system attacks the collagen in the lining of the joints. Scleroderma and morphea are due not to collagen destruction but rather to the overproduction of type I collagen.

At Elaine's next appointment, I was able to give her the good news/bad news. The bad news was that her test results were consistent with a diagnosis of generalized morphea, but this was balanced by the good news that, although she probably had the most severe case I had ever seen, she had no evidence of the dangerous, systemic variant.

"But why me?" she asked plaintively. "Why would I get something like this? Was it something I've done or something I've inherited? And could I have passed this on to my boys?"

"There is no evidence at all that this is an inherited disease, so don't worry about your children. What you have, Elaine, is a rather rare disease, and, to some extent, a mysterious one. We know that when we look under a microscope at the skin of people with morphea, we see a lot of extra collagen, but beyond that, we have a lot to learn about what actually causes it to build up enough to harden the skin."

I could see Elaine was not satisfied, and I wished I could tell her more. But morphea is not a disease with a clear-cut cause like bacteria or viruses, which can be seen under a microscope and killed with antimicrobials. Most researchers now believe that scleroderma is a reaction to some unknown factor or series of events that switch on a gene that programs dermal fibroblasts to synthesize excess collagen, and that the underlying problem is a central one rather than localized to the few apparently affected areas. Most researchers believe the sclerodermas to be another member of the swelling ranks of autoimmune diseases, where the immune system seems to lose its memory selectively and destroys its own tissues as if they were foreign.

The normal immune response is mounted in part by various types of white blood cells and products they produce called *cytokines*. At least a score of different cytokines are involved in coordinating inflammation and other physiologic responses to an invasion by foreign proteins, and more are being identified all the time. One cytokine, called *tumor growth factor beta,* or TGFb, has been shown to be capable of causing collagen-producing cells to proliferate in the dermis. TGFb can be found near the blood vessels of the dermis in patients with scleroderma, but whether it's causing the collagen overproduction emblematic of scleroderma and morphea is still under investigation. An alternate theory maintains that damage to the lining of the blood vessels, particularly small ones, leads to reduced blood flow, which can damage tissues and organs, perhaps triggering the process that leads to excess collagen production.

"So are you telling me there's nothing you can do for me?" Elaine asked.

"No, there are a couple of drugs that might give you some measure of relief."

"Some measure of relief," she cried, "but how much? Am I ever going to look and feel normal again, or am I going to have a lifetime of this horrible skin?"

"Elaine," I said, "I wish we knew more. Nobody has a lot of experience with this disease. I wish I could give you a clear prognosis. In many cases, morphea just goes away by itself. Sometimes that happens after only a few months, and sometimes after a few years. There are a couple of drugs we can try that could help ease the tightness in your skin, but they're quite toxic. There's a drug called D-penicillamine, but its side effects can be worse than the disease. I know it's hard to be asked to be patient when you're having such weird symptoms, but I want to start you on the least toxic therapy first. It's a synthetic corticosteroid cream called Diprolene, and I think it will help. I'd like you to start by putting it just on one side, so that we can see how you respond."

I also explained to Elaine that although her test results almost completely ruled out the possibility of her having systemic disease, her skin symptoms were so severe that I still needed to do further testing to be absolutely certain she did not have any internal involvement.

"But I thought you said my blood tests were negative for systemic problems."

"They are, but you mentioned being unusually constipated for a long time. It's probably just because you're moving around less, but I want to be positive. I'm going to give you the name of a doctor who can do the necessary testing. Don't worry, the tests don't hurt, and they won't take long. The lung function tests involve breathing into an instrument that measures how much air your lungs can hold and how quickly you can empty them. For the esophageal motility tests, you will be given some food containing barium, so the doctor can watch the movements of your esophagus as you swallow."

Elaine left the office looking hopeful. In the hall outside my office as we said good-bye, she gave me the thumbs-up.

I called her a week later to tell her the good news—that the tests had not detected any involvement of her esophagus or lungs.

"Well that's a relief," she said. "I did some reading about scleroderma while I was at the hospital taking the tests. At least I know now I'm not going to die from the kind I have."

When Elaine came in several weeks after that, she seemed mildly cheerful.

"This cream really does seem to be working. I can feel a difference between the areas I'm putting it on and those I'm not. It hasn't helped my back, but maybe that takes time."

Elaine's skin had eased somewhat in the areas where she had applied the cream, although I had hoped for a greater improvement still. I directed her to put the cream on all the affected areas and to return to see me in three weeks.

Elaine was visibly annoyed at our next meeting. "I just want to be well," she said, glaring at me, "and nothing much seems to be happening. I thought the cream was working, but now I think I'm starting to get a new spot on my lower leg, and part of my back is getting worse." She went on to tell me about a magazine article she had read that mentioned a woman with scleroderma. "It said her doctor had given her some new kind of penicillin that helped a lot. Why can't you treat me with that?"

The drug Elaine was referring to was D-penicillamine, a metabolite of penicillin, with no antibiotic properties of its own. It can be useful in morphea and scleroderma, because it prevents the formation of stable bonds among collagen fibers, making newly formed collagen more vulnerable to destruction by the enzyme collagenase. It may also suppress the inappropriate autoimmune response thought to be responsible for the collagen buildup. Although it has been used for thirty years in the treatment of scleroderma, there's still controversy as to its actual efficacy. Theoretically, its direct effect on collagen production should be beneficial. The fact that it is only intermittently so suggests that reliable treatment of morphea may have to wait until someone identifies the gene, or at least the chemical messenger, that carries the erroneous signal to collagen-producing cells and learns how to turn it off.

"I don't mean to question you, but why can't you prescribe it for me?"

"I can, but as I explained to you, I prefer always to start with the safest drugs first. D-penicillamine is still an experimental drug for scleroderma," I told her. "At the moment, the only approved uses of it are for severe, intractable rheumatoid arthritis and certain types of metal poisoning. I wanted to try topical medication first, because D-penicillamine is a very powerful drug with a lot of systemic side effects."

"But if people take it for arthritis, why can't I?"

"If you want to try it, I'm happy to refer you to the scleroderma clinic at the Robert Wood Johnson Medical School, over in New Brunswick, New Jersey," I said. "They're running a study of D-penicillamine there. I'd like to consult with them on your case, since they see many more patients with this disease than I do."

"All right," she said, looking pleased. "I think I'm ready to give it a try. Thank you for letting me have a voice in my treatment. I really appreciate it, even if I'm wrong."

Like many physicians, I am comfortable with patients who take an active interest in their treatment and ask a lot of questions. It's the slightly confrontational patients, in my experience, who often do best at facing down a serious disease.

When the report came back from the scleroderma program in New Brunswick, it confirmed my diagnosis of severe generalized morphea. The doctors there had performed a deeper skin biopsy to rule out eosinophilic fasciitis and had also rerun Elaine's swallowing and lung function tests. The doctor in charge of the research project wrote me that he had seen only fifteen or twenty patients like Elaine over a decade, and, in his experience, such patients were unlikely to improve spontaneously. He recommended starting her on D-penicillamine.

I gave Elaine a prescription for a low-dose regimen of D-penicillamine, with the strict admonition that she return in two weeks so we could check her kidney and liver function, both of which could be severely disrupted by the drug. I told her we would gradually increase her dosage if she didn't experience any side effects, but that since penicillamine loosens all the skin, not just the diseased parts, the rest of her skin could become fragile. We would have to steer the best course we could between hardness and friability.

Once again Elaine and I parted, each hopeful we might make some progress. But when I next saw her, she was again disconsolate.

"I just don't think it's doing any good," she said. I was surprised, since I could see that her skin, particularly on her back, was less rigid than before.

"I still feel like someone has put a straw under my skin and inflated me. The skin on my back is so ugly, I can barely stand to look at it. No man will ever look at me, and even if he did, he wouldn't want to touch me. I'm a misfit. I feel like something in a sideshow. I feel like Turtle Woman!"

Despite what she said, Elaine was better able to move her arms and bend from the waist. Since her blood tests didn't indicate that the D-penicillamine was affecting her liver and kidneys, I decided to increase her dosage slightly. She came in every two weeks for the next three months, and each month I increased her dosage. There was no dramatic improvement, but some of the lesions on her arms appeared to be gradually softening. Even though she was still very uncomfortable, Elaine felt that the treatment was helping.

I was surprised when several months went by and I heard nothing from Elaine. I tried to contact her several times, but to no avail, and she didn't return the telephone messages our staff left on her answering machine. As a last resort, I sent her a certified letter reminding her of penicillamine's toxicity and the urgent need for close supervision if she was still taking the drug.

Then, about six months later, Elaine called and asked to come see me. This time, she was angry.

"That penicillamine stopped working!" she said accusingly. "In fact, it made everything worse. The hard areas still felt like they were encased in Plexiglas, and the rest of my skin was a mess!"

I asked her to explain what she meant.

"All the rest of my skin—the supposedly healthy skin—suddenly went haywire. I was a mass of oozing, raw blisters. One day I scratched an itch on my back, and I tore the skin right off in long strips. It was getting worse, not better. I also had a repulsive metallic taste in my mouth twenty-four hours a day, and my energy level dropped off so much, I could barely drag myself to school. Quite honestly, Dr. Balin, I thought I was dying."

I expressed surprise that she hadn't called me at that point, particularly as I had warned her about the possibility that the drug could affect the healthy parts of her skin in just such a way.

She blushed deeply. "I heard about a doctor in New York who is supposed to know a lot about scleroderma. He said my symptoms were a typical reaction to penicillamine and that I should stop taking it immediately. I did, and the soreness and the rawness cleared up, but then the tightness came right back." She looked me in the eye and then burst into tears. "I'm sorry. I didn't mean to second-guess you. I've been so embarrassed even to come back here. Isn't there anything you can do for me? I just don't think I can cope anymore." Tears streaked down her cheeks.

When people are confronted with the kind of rare and mysterious disease Elaine has, they are understandably furious when no one can give them a definite prognosis or a treatment that works magic. Many of them do exactly what Elaine started to do: they go from doctor to doctor, hoping to hear an answer they can live with.

We don't yet understand what makes the scarring process go wild in morphea and scleroderma, and so we have no treatment that goes to the root of the problem. We only have therapies that attack the problem somewhere farther downstream. Most doctors agree that one of the saddest aspects of our profession is that we can't restore all patients to a state of perfect or even functional health. Sometimes the best we can do is keep them from getting worse. Yet this is understandably difficult for most patients to accept. Their reverence for medical science is so great that if it falls short when they most need it, they feel they have been singled out.

"Elaine, I have no problem with your having gotten another opinion. It's just that I was worried for you. If you want to work with me, we'll continue to explore every possible treatment, but you have to promise you won't disappear again without talking to me first. These are strong medications I am treating you with, and you have to be followed closely."

"All right," she said. "I'm with you."

"There is another drug we could try. There's less in the literature about using it in scleroderma, but it also has fewer side effects than penicillamine."

"What is it?"

"It's called Plaquenil. It was developed to treat resistant cases of malaria. Now I want to stress again that we're entering fairly uncharted waters with this. It's a relatively safe drug, but it may not do a thing for you. You'll need to have an eye exam before you start and every six months thereafter, and we'll still need to run periodic blood tests." I decided to prescribe another topical steroid ointment that might help make her skin feel better and suggested she also apply Eucerin, an over-the-counter lotion, to help combat the dryness.

As I watched Elaine leave my office, it occurred to me that perhaps she was going to be one of the frustrating patients I couldn't help. One of my friends once said to me that I must like the most mysterious cases best, because they must bring out the researcher in me. But the truth is that I prefer patients I can actually do something concrete to help.

Elaine's case was a tough one, because of the rarity and general lack of understanding of morphea and because of the extensiveness of her involvement. As a corollary, I can think of other patients whose problems seem utterly ordinary—except that I can't cure them. For example, at the moment I am trying to treat a patient who has developed a diabolical case of hives. Certainly, hives are a common enough symptom. But therein lies the problem: what are they symptoms *of*? I can't figure out what's causing them, even though I've been seeing this man for several months. Although I can give him skin creams that somewhat soothe his eruptions, I don't know why the hives are appearing in the first place. I'm the fourth doctor this poor man has seen, and I'd do anything to help him. He's a young, married father of three. Because of his skin problem he's been out of work for six months, and his disability is due to run out in a couple of weeks.

Cases like his and Elaine's distress me. I don't like putting people through the hunting and pecking for the right treatment. They get frustrated, and so do I. I want to be able to cure them and send them back into their lives. When a patient comes in with cancer, I know what to do. I remove the cancer, and I've cured the problem. I am not particularly fond of cases that are so difficult I can't solve them for patients. I feel inadequate, as though I've gotten a math problem wrong. Even in cases where there may be no answer known to medical science I feel I *should* be able to solve the problem. Of course, in a perfect world, where I had endless time, I could take all these recalcitrant problems on as research projects and really get into them. But because my time is finite and I can't make a whole study of every patient with a difficult problem, I have to reserve what time is left over from my practice for my research into the biochemical basis of the aging process. I know this is the way I can help the greatest number of people. Yet how can I explain that to a patient whose entire life has been reduced to a symptom?

After Elaine had been taking the Plaquenil for six weeks, we both agreed her skin was better, particularly on her back. Instead of its being as hard as fiberglass to the touch, I was able to move it gently with my fingers.

Back in my office, Elaine told me that she had recently begun attending a support group for scleroderma patients run by a nationwide group called the Scleroderma Federation.

"It's taken me months to get up the courage to do this," she said. "I was terrified of what I might see there. I was afraid, I guess, that I might be looking at my own future. But when I finally went, it was terrific. The people were so upbeat, and I realized how much I've needed to talk about this with someone who knows exactly what I'm going through."

She told me of a new study she had heard about at a meeting that would evaluate the use of a therapy called photopheresis. (Pheresis is a procedure whereby blood is withdrawn from a patient, a particular type of blood cell is retained, treated, and reinfused into the patient.) In this case, T lymphocytes, the white blood cells that essentially command one wing of our immune response, are separated out, treated with a drug that makes them sensitive to light, then exposed to ultraviolet light, which destroys some of their ability to do their job. In the case of scleroderma, the goal is to suppress the immune system sufficiently so that it can't turn against the body's connective tissue. Although I knew this approach was being tried in scleroderma, I was most familiar with it in the treatment of mycosis fungoides, the same type of T cell cancer that Loretta's troubled adolescent patient, Trish Simons, was suffering from.

"I think it's certainly worth exploring, if you'd like to try it. Chances are it's a double-blind study, and you won't be certain whether you are being treated or given a placebo," I warned.

"I'll take that chance," she said. "The person who told me about it at the group said this treatment supposedly made people's skin a lot better."

We decided to continue Elaine's Plaquenil dosage at the same level while I explored the possibility of her entering the photopheresis study.

As it turned out, Elaine was ineligible for the study, which was restricted to patients with systemic involvement. I decided to wait until her next appointment to break the news to her. She had pinned her hopes on this particular answer to her problem, and I wanted to make sure her disappointment didn't lead her to abandon the Plaquenil while she went off in search of another ready answer.

About a week before Elaine was due to come in for a visit, Loretta and I were sitting in our library, with a stack of new journals between us. The fact that we share the same profession adds a dimension of intellectual pleasure to our marriage that I cannot imagine being without. To sit with her after supper has been cleared, talking about our patients, planning experiments, or just reading, is, for me, the essence of marital contentment. Alas, with our busy schedules, it is all too rare a pleasure.

Toward the end of the evening, I was just about to close the journal I was reading when a brief letter to the editor, under the headline "Morphea and Anti-Hypertensive Therapy," caught my eye. In the letter, a dermatologist reported having seen three cases of morphea that developed in patients who had taken a commonly prescribed blood pressure pill for many years. He did not propose any explanation. He was merely reporting an association, but it was enough to set my mind racing. I passed the journal over to Loretta, who had put down her own stack of journals in favor of a novel.

"My morphea patient, Elaine Howard, has been taking an anti-hypertensive for at least ten years," I said.

"Do you remember which one she's taking?"

"I'll have to look at her chart in the morning."

"Who knows what reports like this mean," Loretta said, clearly unimpressed by the small number of cases. "Do you remember that dentist I treated for morphea? His wasn't nearly as extensive or as long-standing as Elaine's, but he was convinced he had gotten it after taking erythromycin for an infection. By the time he had made the association, his lesions had responded to Diprolene, so we never figured out whether he was right or not."

Every physician can think of cases in which a patient decides his or her symptoms are due to a particular drug or to eating meat or environmental exposure, avoids the suspected trigger, and the symptoms vanish, only to return when the offending food or drug is reintroduced. Rarely can the truth of the patient's hunch be proven or disproven, yet the "cure" is indisputable. There is still so much to learn about the roles of suggestion and belief in healing. Some physicians speak dismissively of the "placebo effect" as though any cure not effected through conventional medical means is somehow invalid. To my way of thinking, the ability to marshal the placebo effect is an important facet, albeit a mysterious one, of the healer's art.

The next morning, I checked Elaine's chart and found she was indeed taking the drug mentioned in the letter. I knew I must proceed cautiously when suggesting to Elaine that changing her blood pressure medication might help her skin symptoms. She was so vulnerable and so easily disappointed. It was entirely possible that the change of medication would have no effect, and I was afraid she might, once again, depart in despair. She had been showing slow improvement on the Plaquenil, and no new patches of morphea had developed recently. I was reluctant to compromise her progress on the basis of an anecdotal report, but the severity of her disease mandated my trying everything.

"Elaine," I began, "I've been doing some reading about the newest research in your disease. There have been a couple of cases reported in which people taking the drug Tenormin for high blood pressure have developed hardening of the skin. To be honest, I don't know what to make of this, because the association hasn't been thoroughly studied. Even so, I'm going to suggest that you switch to another antihypertensive for a few months."

"Dr. Balin, I'll try anything," Elaine replied wearily. "I just want to get better."

Elaine Howard was jubilant when she arrived in my office for her next checkup a month later. Without her even saying a word, I could sense that her spirits had lifted. I realized I had never seen Elaine smile before, but now her pretty blue eyes radiated delight.

"Dr. Balin, I can't wait for you to examine me!" she said, her smile flooding her face.

When I entered the examining room, she was pacing the floor, a decided contrast to the frightened, disconsolate patient who usually huddled on my examining table.

"Take a look at my stomach," she said. But before I could do so, she grabbed a small roll of flesh and began to knead it vigorously. "Look, loose skin! No more 'can't pinch an inch' on me."

Indeed, the skin on her stomach, which had been waxy and rigid only weeks before, was now becoming pliant and soft.

"I never thought jiggly skin would make me so happy." She laughed. "This is the best part, but look at my back, look at my arms. It's all getting better. I'm on my way! And you know what? The constipation is gone too. Literally overnight. I know no one thought I had systemic involvement, but I was never constipated until this all started in my skin, and now it's gone."

"Your skin is definitely better. There's no question," I averred cautiously.

"Oh, I know I'm not out of the woods yet, but at least I feel like a human again. I'm back inside my own body instead of a turtle's."

Over the months that followed, Elaine's skin continued to soften. After the initial burst of improvement, the changes were more gradual, but Elaine was clearly getting better.

"Look," she said to me one day, holding up her arms and clapping her hands so I could see the loose flesh swinging from her arms. "The applause muscle! I never thought I'd be happy to see *that* come back, but am I ever. You know what else? I'm finding I have to turn the heat up in my apartment, because I'm not living inside a turtle shell anymore."

Morphea, like all the autoimmune diseases, is an enigma.

Whether it was in fact the change in her medication that began her transformation or whether the signal that was instructing her fibroblasts to go awry had started to die down would be impossible to say for certain. I still see Elaine every few months. Her morphea has receded, and although there is some residual hardness and scarring deep in her skin, Elaine is no longer trapped inside a carapace.

Of Time and the Skin

〰️ ∽⊘∾ 〰️

"Play me a nocturne, Dorian, and as you play, tell me in a low voice how you have kept your youth. You must have some secret. I am only ten years older than you are, and I am wrinkled, and worn and yellow."

OSCAR WILDE,
THE PICTURE OF DORIAN GRAY

"**D**r. Pratt, no matter what a male patient thinks about being examined by a woman, there is no room for modesty in the practice of dermatology!" The voice of Dr. George Hambrick, the department chairman during my first year of residency at New York Hospital, wafted back into my mind several years later as I glimpsed the name of my next patient in the clinic appointment book. "I don't care if it's President Reagan himself and he's showing you a wart on the palm of his hand," he continued in his distinguished southern accent. "He's still got to take his clothes off and let you examine every square millimeter of his skin with a light and a magnifier. It's not optional!" He was delivering this lecture in response to my failure to evaluate the entire body surface of a very shy college student, only a few years younger than I, who had come in for removal of a cluster of painful plantar warts on the sole of one foot. The student had objected strenuously to a full skin survey, and since his complaint was localized and he seemed to be otherwise in perfect health, I decided not to insist on exploring his entire body for any lurking pathology. Of course, we had been taught in medical school that even if a person presented with a complaint limited to one square inch of skin, we should always assess first-time patients from head to toe and take a complete history. Yet in this case, admittedly one of my earliest unsupervised medical encounters with a dermatology patient, the young man's awkwardness fed into my own inexperience and managed to overwhelm the best instincts of the trained doctor with seven years of medical education behind her.

After Dr. Hambrick had left the floor, the attending physician, who had overheard our chief's remarks, turned to me with the old medical school saw: "Don't ever forget, Dr. Pratt, that if you hear hoofbeats, chances are it's only a horse, but you'd better look hard, because it might just be a zebra." Then he went on to tell me his version of every young doctor's worst nightmare: "My first week, I saw a little old lady with dishwater dermatitis on her hands. What I didn't see was the melanoma on her back, because I didn't want to embarrass her by asking her to undress completely. When she came back for a checkup three weeks later, she was seen by the chief resident, and guess what? Surprise, surprise!"

That incident had taken place several years earlier. Now I was in my third year of residency and quite sure of myself. Nevertheless, the modesty issue had momentarily resurfaced in the person of Sister Elizabeth, my next patient, a nun from a convent in New Jersey. I did not grow up around nuns, and to me they seemed to represent womanhood at its shyest and least natural. Was I going to have a problem convincing this woman, whose religion dictated that she keep her body covered and who presumably was therefore uncomfortable with the flesh, to stand nearly naked in front of me while I examined her every pore with a light and magnifier?

Just as Sister Elizabeth and I had made our introductions, my telephone rang. It was the laboratory, with some results on another patient. As I sat on hold, waiting to speak with the dermatopathologist, I took in what I could of Sister Elizabeth. Judging by the small square of leathery, sallow skin not covered by her wimple, and by her hands, which looked as though she were wearing pigskin gloves, I guessed her to be in her late sixties.

"I'm forty-nine," she replied in answer to the first question of her medical history. Even with all the sophisticated measuring devices, scales, and questionnaires available to modern medicine, nothing is more accurate in estimating chronologic age than the human eye. Yet in order to make an accurate judgment of a person's age, a great deal of visual information must be synthesized instantaneously. In Sister Elizabeth's case, I was blinded to most of the necessary cues by her habit. My judgment was perforce based on a small area of sun-exposed skin.

As we chatted about Sister Elizabeth's life, I learned that she had entered the convent at age twenty. She worked in the convent's office and ran a local center for troubled adolescents. In addition, she spent many hours a week outdoors.

"I do enjoy gardening, and I think I'm pretty good at it," she admitted with evident pride.

"Why are you here today, Sister Elizabeth?" I asked.

"I decided to come because of these two spots on the left side of my nose," she said. "I can feel them when I wash my face, and they feel like sandpaper. I just wanted to make sure they weren't a problem."

"I'll need to look at them under the magnifier," I told her cautiously. "I will also want to check the rest of your skin." I wondered whether there was some protocol or etiquette to a nun's disrobing. "Why don't you put on this gown and just knock on the door for me when you're ready?" I left the room.

"Thank you," she said, taking the flimsy garment everyone dislikes.

Soon after I was seated at my desk in the adjoining office, she knocked. It hardly seemed long enough for her to have removed all her robes. I hoped she hadn't misunderstood. But when I entered the examining room, she was correctly attired, with no evidence of embarrassment as she turned to me. (Over years, I have noticed that the nuns I have treated seem to suffer none of the embarrassment at disrobing that many of my patients do. I have often wondered whether this is because they do not typically view the human body in a sexual context.)

"What a lovely view of the river from here," she said as I took in the figure confronting me.

Although the skin not covered by her wimple belied her true age, the rest of her face suggested the twenty-year-old supplicant who had entered the convent a quarter of a lifetime earlier. Side by side with skin that showed signs of aging was skin that appeared ageless. Here stood a personification of what some of the new research was revealing.

Although most people think of time as having a detrimental effect on the skin, it is not time alone but rather the combination of time and the external milieu that most ravages our surfaces. It is the accumulation of depredations by sun, wind, low-humidity indoor environments, and various chemical irritants that produces most of the cutaneous stigmata almost universally associated with aging. Heredity dictates the skin's susceptibility to the elements and its ability to repair itself, and gravity and chemical changes within the skin also take their toll. But if environmental ravages were subtracted from the picture, many people in their nineties could have the velvety integument of youth.

I put on my magnifiers and examined Sister Elizabeth. Aside from the two spots she had mentioned and two more I found, her skin was unremarkable. The average individual has about ten moles, and Sister Elizabeth had her full complement of these, but none looked in the least threatening or worthy of biopsying. I turned my attention to her face to look more closely at the four small pinkish plaques on either side of her nose.

"How long do you think you've had these spots, Sister Elizabeth?"

"Doctor, I'm not sure. It must sound odd to a pretty girl like you, but I don't see myself in the mirror very often. Dr. Webb told me I had them a couple of months ago, so I know it's been at least that long."

"What you have is very common," I assured her. "There are two possibilities. They could be actinic keratoses, or they could be small, early skin cancers. We do need to biopsy them to find out which they are, but in either case there is nothing to worry about. Why don't you get dressed and come into my office next door when you're ready, and we'll talk about where we go from here."

In my office, I took out a mirror and showed Sister Elizabeth the spots under a magnifying glass I held up to her face. "This is what we're talking about. Actinic keratoses are referred to as precancerous lesions, but that's not really an accurate description. What we're looking at are cancerous cells that haven't gone anywhere. They're still in the upper layer of the skin. They might not develop any further, or they might grow down into the skin. Some of these things go on and transform into a type of cancer called squamous cell carcinoma."

"That does sound serious," she said. The gentle smile that had played across her face for most of her visit was now shadowed by worry.

"Skin cancers are very common, mostly in people who have had quite a bit of sun exposure. I would hazard a guess that any problems of this type that you ever have will be either in the area of your face that is not protected by your wimple or on your hands."

I noticed a slight nervous tremor in her voice as she said, "All right, what do we do to get started?"

Before proceeding, I explained exactly what I would do, reassuring her that there would be no discomfort. I injected a local anesthetic near the lesions, then gently shaved a tiny piece off each lesion and placed them in a bottle of fixative for transport to the dermatopathology lab at Cornell, where they would be examined. Although she didn't articulate it, I knew she was worried about how long she would have to wait for the results. I said, "We'll have the biopsy report in four or five days. In the meantime, don't worry. Once we have the results, we can discuss the various treatment options."

Around this time, the heads of the lab at Rockefeller where I worked as part of my residency training—Dr. Arthur Balin, and Dr. Martin Carter—were starting a study in their laboratory of investigative dermatology. They wanted to examine the effects of trans-retinoic acid, a vitamin A–derived compound, on actinic keratoses and other types of sun damage. Although Retin-A had been used to treat acne for many years prior to this, it was still an experimental treatment for these other skin problems. In order to recruit patients, they had placed several advertisements in the *New York Times* and local newspapers. Sister Elizabeth seemed to me to present a unique and valuable research subject, for she, in effect, could act as her own control. I had no idea whether it would even be possible for her to participate, but I decided to pose the question.

"Sister Elizabeth, in addition to my work here, I also work next door at Rockefeller University, where we are studying a new type of medication for the treatment of skin lesions such as yours. Because you do spend so much time outdoors, there is some chance of your developing more of these spots in the future. I think this drug might be valuable to you. We believe that it might actually reverse many precancerous changes. And, as a side benefit, many patients are finding that it makes their skin look younger." As I looked at the sun-damaged skin in the center of her face and thought of what lay beneath her wimple, I thought of the Chinese yin-yang symbol. I yearned to return that ravaged skin to the pristine state of the rest of her face. I knew I couldn't repair it perfectly, but I could make a major improvement. It was one of the most interesting challenges I had so far encountered in the practice of my chosen specialty.

"It would be fascinating to be part of a research project, but I'm not sure I want to look younger," she said, laughing. "I don't mean to seem ungrateful, but you see, to me, lines are beautiful. Think of Mother Teresa or Robert Frost. I don't view them as ugly. Every line on those faces means something. In my case, my wrinkles mean something happy—all those lovely hours with my plants."

I felt foolish and superficial. I tried not to blush. Of course Sister Elizabeth, who didn't dwell on her external image, would have a more accepting view of the cutaneous signs of aging. Part of me agreed with her. I find expression lines around the eyes and mouth attractive to look at, because I know they come from smiling, whereas I find smoker's lines in the upper lip and sun-related blotchiness and broken blood vessels especially unattractive. I was so used to patients for whom any sign of aging was a horror, something to be disguised and avoided. I envied Sister Elizabeth her ability to live life without a thought about her appearance. That probably *was* the will of our Creator. I wished I had been less quick to mention what was the least significant of Retin-A's benefits. I struggled to explain myself.

"Sister Elizabeth, I understand your feelings, and to some extent I share them," I said. "But as a dermatologist, I have been taught to distinguish between normal aging and environmental damage. To the average eye they are one and the same, but they really are not. The skin at the center of your face, where these lesions have appeared, is wounded skin." In my eagerness to get her into the study, I wanted to say, "This is not what God intended for your skin." But I knew this would probably sound somewhat pompous. Instead, I decided to let the whole issue drop until our next appointment, when I would have the path report in hand.

The report that came back a few days later indicated Sister Elizabeth's problem could easily be taken care of. Her lesions were precancerous actinic keratoses and not full-fledged cancers. Nevertheless, they needed treatment.

Although I could have removed Sister Elizabeth's actinic keratoses by dermabrasion, by applying a chemical peel that would slough off the top layer of skin, or with 5-fluorouracil, a topical chemotherapeutic agent, she and I decided to freeze the spots with liquid nitrogen. This method, the one most commonly used, is fast, although not entirely painless. I tell patients it feels like having an ice cube and a match on their skin at the same time. Nevertheless, most people tolerate it without a local anesthetic. Sister Elizabeth was not concerned that this method might leave a white spot behind.

At the risk of sounding insistent, I thought I would remind her of our discussion about the Retin-A study.

"Sister Elizabeth, do you remember that at your last appointment we talked about your participation in a research project we are conducting?"

"Of course," she replied, her face pleasant as ever but impassive.

"You've had some sun damage that requires attention. Even though sun damage may look to most people like normal aging, there are some important differences. One is natural and gradual, and the other is a medical problem that shouldn't be ignored. We think this new drug shows real promise in treating the type of precancerous growths you have and in preventing more from forming in areas that have been sun damaged."

"I would be very interested in volunteering for your study if you think this treatment would be helpful," she said.

"I have to explain that this is what is called a double-blind study. Half the patients will be randomly selected to receive Retin-A, and half will be given a placebo treatment. Neither the patients nor the physicians involved in the study will know who is receiving the real treatment. So there is only a fifty-fifty chance that you will actually be getting the active drug. But if you don't get it and the study suggests a benefit, you'll be given the opportunity later to be treated with it."

Although I had my volunteer, I wanted to make certain she really understood what was, at that time, a new concept in dermatology. Researchers were just beginning to explore the differences between aging and environmental damage.

I explained to her that the normal intrinsic aging of skin, without factoring in the effects of sun exposure, is a continual process that begins in our twenties. As early as the middle of that decade, we begin to lose collagen, the structural protein matrix that gives the skin body and strength. Although collagen begins to disappear from the skin at the rate of about 1 percent per year, sun exposure can greatly hasten this process. Skin not protected from UV radiation is actually in a constant state of mild inflammation. (Nowadays, when Arthur's and my patients insist that their skin looks more youthful to them when they have a tan, we explain that this chronic mild inflammation makes the skin swell slightly, plumping up fine lines and causing the skin to reflect more light, both of which lend a more youthful appearance.) In addition to its deleterious effects on collagen, the sun also attacks elastin. Although the number of elastic fibers normally decreases throughout adult life, it does so in massive increments in sun-damaged skin. Moreover, the fibers lose their normal architecture and degenerate into a tangled, disorganized mass, like a ball made from elastic bands. Solar radiation also damages small blood vessels in the skin, to the point where many disappear, decreasing the flow of blood and nutrients to the skin.

By the time we reach our thirties, the skin becomes less resilient as elastic tissue continues to be lost. This loss of resilience allows gravity to begin to have its way. Drooping and sagging may become apparent even in relatively pristine skin. Unlike other parts of the body, in which muscles are attached to ligaments or tendons, which connect them to bones, the facial muscles are attached directly to the skin. Every time these muscles are used, a groove forms beneath the skin. (This is why facial exercises, which once formed a separate chapter in every exercise book and magazine article about maintaining a youthful appearance, are now known to accomplish just the opposite and are no longer advocated.) As elasticity continues to diminish—either slowly, as a result of normal aging, or more rapidly, due to solar damage—the skin, in effect, loses its memory and becomes less able to snap back. Repetitive movements, such as those performed in order to frown, squint, or hold a cigarette between the lips, form the first permanent wrinkles. In many Asian societies, where people are taught to maintain a poker face, these wrinkles don't form, and it's often hard to determine people's ages from their faces.

As we age, creases due to habitual sleeping positions begin to appear. This is because the fat pad that plumps up our skin like the stuffing of an upholstered chair begins to disappear, leaving behind pouches that exacerbate the effects of our already stretched-out fabric. These vertical rays on the cheeks and forehead can be prevented if we sleep on our backs to prevent the skin from crumpling against the pillow.

Around this time, the process by which new cells are constantly being born in the lower layers of the epidermis and then pushed up through the epidermis slows down. Instead of renewing itself every twenty-eight days or so, as it does in youth, the top layer of the skin takes longer to shed. The process itself may become disorganized, with cells clumping together. For this reason, our skin tends to look duller, drier, and scalier as we age. Exfoliating regimens, ranging from a brisk rub with a washcloth or Buf-Puf to alpha-hydroxy acids and Retin-A, work in part by speeding up the shedding of these old, dead cells.

Normal aging changes become even more apparent in the fifth decade of life. The combination of gravity, the pull of the facial muscles, and collagen changes contribute to deeper expression lines and furrows around the nose and mouth. The loss of skin elasticity is ever more apparent. Around this age, people begin to find that weight loss is a double-edged sword. While their bodies may look and feel better as they shed pounds, their faces may age radically following a significant weight loss, because the unsupported skin doesn't rebound as it did when it was more elastic. One good reason to deal with weight loss early in life is that before age thirty-five, the skin should have enough elasticity to take up the slack. Afterward it may not, depending upon how much environmental damage has already occurred. When I describe this process to my patients, it recalls to me a line from *Henry IV, Part I,* in which Falstaff says to Bardolph, "Why, my skin hangs about me like an old lady's loose gown; I am withered like an old apple-john."

The intrinsic aging process accelerates in the fifties. The skin's elasticity drops off sharply, leaving it even more prey to the constant presence of gravity. Gravity also causes the tip of the nose to droop and the ears to elongate. At menopause, and somewhat later in men, the resorption of bone speeds up. As the bones shrink away from the skin, the skin retains its size and shape, so that it is slightly bigger than the underlying bones. It is actually this loss of bony support and some of the overlying fat pad that results in the loose folds of skin and thick wrinkles that many people develop at this time. This is another reason, I explain to my patients, why it's so important to ensure healthy bones by getting enough calcium and avoiding smoking. Many women who are fairly blithe about the possibility of developing osteoporosis as they age take the threat of sagging skin far more seriously. I often think it's an approach that more doctors should take when urging these lifestyle changes, rather than merely warning their patients about the risk of fractures several decades in their future. Eventually bone loss will cause the chin to fall. Changes in the teeth and jaw also contribute to the collapse of the lower part of the face.

Continuing to describe these changes to Sister Elizabeth, I assured her they are normal. "Doesn't the sun just speed up the natural aging process?" Sister Elizabeth asked. "Don't all those things you've described happen, but happen sooner?"

"Some people think ultraviolet damage is just an accelerated version of normal aging, but the two processes seem to be quite different on a microscopic level, even if they look the same to the naked eye."

The relationship between intrinsic aging and photoaging continues to be disputed. There are enough areas of overlap to make us uncertain about whether the two processes are truly different. One possible bridge between them could involve free radicals.

Free radicals are highly unstable oxygen molecules. They can be considered normal in that they are constantly being generated as the body goes about its business of using oxygen. However, smoking, dietary factors, and sunlight can also generate free radicals, which add to the body's burden. Free radicals are extremely reactive, because they must find electrons of other atoms to join up with in order to achieve stabilization. Once this occurs, a chain reaction of sorts begins, as a result of which thousands of other free radicals are formed. Free radicals can harm cells in many ways. They are able to damage the genetic machinery of the cell, and they can react with the cell membrane, theoretically impairing a cell's ability to respond to hormones or altering its permeability to various molecules. Fortunately, our body has many built-in mechanisms for neutralizing free radicals. For instance, several enzymes seem to offer some protection, and mechanisms within the cells trap free radicals so they can't harm important cellular structures. Melanin, the pigment in our skin, protects against sunlight-induced free-radical damage by acting as a free-radical trap.

One theory of photoaging is that it represents a degree of damage that would never be seen in sun-protected skin over a normal human life span. If, however, that same protected skin could be studied after five hundred years, the same changes that come with ultraviolet damage in as few as thirty years might then be visible, because both may be linked to the accumulation of free-radical damage. In sun-protected skin, the damage would accumulate more slowly than in skin constantly being bombarded by free-radical-generating sunlight. It can perhaps be said that in this way, photodamage represents an acceleration of the normal aging process. Sunlight is simply an additional source of free-radical damage. The sunscreens available to us today protect us against the immediate burning caused by ultraviolet B rays, but most offer little protection against the destruction of elastic tissue and pigment changes caused by UVA light. And sunscreens are just beginning to be developed to help protect us from free-radical damage, which may turn out to be the most harmful aspect of suntanning.

After I had summarized this complicated research as best I could for Sister Elizabeth, she stood up and said, "Well, I don't want to keep you here all day answering questions when you have patients to see." Sister Elizabeth was clearly eager to go, and we said good-bye.

What I might have continued to tell her is that sun damage is cumulative and remains hidden to the naked eye for decades. This fact complicates Arthur's and my job, since it permits sun worshipers to continue tanning with a false sense of impunity. In fact, it is estimated that nearly 80 percent of the sun damage to the skin occurs by age eighteen. Even people who don't set out to get a tan may accumulate significant sun exposure if they merely go about their daily lives without thinking or remembering to protect themselves. Forty years of hanging the laundry, sitting in the bleachers at Little League games and walking on the sunny side of the street without protection can be enough to cause wrinkles, various types of spots and lesions, and even cancers in certain skin types. I see such patients every day.

I was particularly excited by the prospect of having Sister Elizabeth in the Retin-A study, for even though the study itself was restricted to evaluating the effect of Retin-A or a placebo in the treatment of actinic keratoses and sun damage, she herself was a unique laboratory. Although observations have been made of the skin of Tibetan monks who enter the monastery in their early teens and spend the rest of their lives in contemplation, their faces unsullied by emotion and rarely touched by daylight, such artificial circumstances permit us to view only how the skin behaves under these most rarefied conditions. We learn from them about the pure effects of time and gravity.

Most other studies of intrinsic aging have been performed on skin normally kept clothed, like that of the inner upper arm or buttocks. Findings from these studies are also of limited value in helping us tease apart the effects of photoaging and normal aging, because the skin is not a single-issue fabric upholstering our entire body. The enormous variations in thickness, hair cover, texture, and blood supply render comparisons between facial skin and that on any other area only partially useful. Furthermore, these areas lack the face's unique ability to form itself into expressions. No scientist could have hoped for a neater, more parsimonious experiment than Sister Elizabeth's face, with its adjacent areas of virgin facial skin and identical skin with an overlay of solar damage.

Not long after my first meetings with Sister Elizabeth, another patient contacted us about participating in the study. Unlike Sister Elizabeth, Hillary was most anxious to partake of Retin-A's putative anti-aging effect.

Hillary King had the muscular presence and physical grace that bespeak trained bodies—those of athletes and dancers. Tall and very slim, she had natural topaz-blonde hair that hung to her shoulders in thick festoons. She was carefully made-up, but even the custom-blended foundation was powerless to cover her extremely weathered complexion. Studying her as she introduced herself, I wondered how she spent her time—her skin was so ravaged. Even from the social distance at which I stood, I could see mats of broken capillaries on her nose and cheeks. Hidden among her many freckles and liver spots were a number of suspicious-looking areas that demanded a biopsy. Her entire face was crosshatched with fine lines, like cobwebs across her face, and her upper lip was scored with the typical purse-string wrinkles of the heavy smoker. Although her skin told me that she was in her late fifties, her overall gestalt suggested she was probably at least fifteen or even twenty years younger.

"If you're wondering how old I am, I'm not as old as I look." Her bourbon-brown eyes blinked hard. These patients who wisecracked to cover their feelings were often those who most wanted my help and yet didn't want to admit how deeply their appearance upset them. "Actually, I just turned forty last week," she said, her voice growing brittle.

Hillary King, it turned out, was an accomplished equestrian, an Olympic hopeful who had already represented the United States at several major international competitions. "I don't want to sound like I'm boasting," she said, fixing me in her intense gaze, "but I am one of the top riders in the country. I show, I coach, I judge, and I am outdoors all day long. In the winters, I teach and compete on the Florida circuit."

"Married? Children?" I asked.

"Engaged and about to be a stepmother," she said, her face softening. "And that's why I hope you can fix me up."

"I'll certainly do my best," I said. The damage was so severe, I couldn't help but wonder how effective Retin-A would be for her. She was really a candidate for more major work. "Do you sunbathe a lot?" I queried.

"No! I don't sunbathe at all. I'd never have time. I'm in the barn riding and teaching about ten hours a day, and it's been like that since high school," she replied indignantly. "I just go about my life, but it all takes place in the sun. I get sun on my face and arms, as you can see, but the rest of my body is as white as a fish belly." She held up her hands, which were surprisingly pale appendages to her bronzed arms. I thought back to Sister Elizabeth's hands, which had reminded me of pigskin gloves. Hillary's looked more like white kid.

"Gloves," she said. "I never ride without gloves."

"Do you use a sunscreen?" I asked, although the answer was obvious.

"No, as you can see, I have not been using any. I didn't see the point of glomming on all that grease, which I just sweat off after twenty minutes of riding anyway. I like to be tan—or at least I did, until I found out what came later."

"When did you first notice changes in your skin?"

"I guess it was after David and I started getting serious. I mean, I'm sure they were there before that, but I wasn't really scrutinizing my skin. He's the first man I've gone out with in years who isn't a rider, and he's also a bit younger than I am, which makes me nervous. I think there are two kinds of women: those who go out with older men because they feel younger in comparison, and those who go out with younger men because they feel young along with them. I always used to like older men, so I had no problem. One day it just hit me that David and I might eventually become one of those depressing couples where the woman looks like a wrinkled old battle-ax and everyone assumes her husband is her son."

At home one evening, she had sat in front of one of those mirrors with a magnifier on one side and taken stock of what her face had become.

"I was horrified by what I saw. I'm not particularly vain. I've always done my best to look attractive—which used to mean clean hair, a great tan, and maybe a little lipstick. Sitting there, forcing myself to look hard, I realized that strangers weren't seeing me the way I thought I looked. It made me sad for David especially. I wanted to be 'that pretty girl David married,' and I realized that night it was probably too late. Sure, I could still be 'that nice woman David married' or 'that wife of David's who's riding in the Olympics,' but never *pretty* anymore. The next morning, I went to a department store and bought up every skin cream the Lancôme people told me to buy, and then I found an even more expensive counter, where they made me some custom foundation that I now wear every minute I'm not on a horse. Unfortunately, it doesn't really cover the mess I've made of my face."

I felt so sorry for her. So many women of her age were beginning to come in with skin very much like hers. "Well, weren't we all supposed to be 'California Girls,' like that stupid song?" one of them once said to me. When they were growing up, the only summer beauty advice that the magazines mustered up counseled readers about how to get a better tan faster and how to keep it longer. By the time the media had begun to relay the dermatologists' warnings about tanning, many women of Hillary's age already had the skin of women a decade older.

"I realize this is all old hat to you," Hillary said. "You're probably sitting there thinking what an idiot I am to have fried my skin and then come back and ask for a second chance."

"No, I was thinking about how to give you that second chance." Hillary wasn't asking for a second chance so much as the chance to begin a second act in a life that had been dedicated to achieving difficult goals. That was certainly a need I could empathize with after eight years of medical education, two residencies, and a research fellowship.

"I feel kind of helpless. I'm used to getting on twelve-hundred-pound horses and training them to do as I ask. I'm used to being in control, and it seems that I can't control my skin—at all. I can't even hide it. I mean, you can go to the gym if your body starts to betray you, you can dye your hair if it's going gray, but your face. . . . What can you do to fix a face like this?" She looked at me imploringly and sighed. "I never really thought about the future. I never expected my skin could look like this so soon, and I never used to think I'd care when it finally did."

Hillary's pathology report came back with a diagnosis of two basal cell cancers and two actinic keratoses—too few to qualify her for the Retin-A study.

"I'm sorry to disappoint you about the study," I told her over the telephone. "You have only two of the precancerous growths that we are looking at in the trial, but you do have a couple of skin cancers of a type called basal cell carcinomas that need to be removed at your convenience."

"But does that mean I can't try Retin-A?" she asked, disappointment cramping her voice.

"I can still treat you in my office, and that way you can be certain of getting active Retin-A. In the study, you'd have an equal chance of getting a placebo instead."

"I don't have the bad kind of skin cancer, do I?"

"No, you don't have a melanoma. This kind of skin cancer has a high cure rate, and basal cell cancers do not generally spread to other parts of the body."

"Are you sure?" she asked nervously.

"Not as long as they are recognized and treated early. Basal cell cancers do not usually metastasize, but they can spread locally. Squamous cell cancers can metastasize, but even that's uncommon unless they are neglected."

Basal cell cancers are spawned in the foundation, or basal, layer of the epidermis. As skin lesions go, they usually appear nondescript—certainly not ominous-looking things that would say *cancer* to the average person. Patients who have picked at or shaved around a little spot for years are often incredulous when a diagnosis of a basal cell cancer is made. A small sore, like a perpetually nascent pimple, a scab that comes and goes, a flat, pearly area, or even just a persistent dry area—these innocent manifestations are easy to misinterpret or ignore.

I explained to Hillary that the flat, slightly crusty spot on her cheek was an actinic keratosis, which could turn into a squamous cell cancer, a slightly less common form of skin cancer. Squamous cell cancers are almost always emblematic of sun damage and frequently arise from an existing solar keratosis. Like basal cell cancers, squamous cell cancers are highly curable if detected and treated soon enough. This was before Arthur had taken his training in Mohs micrographic surgery. Nowadays I refer all my patients with skin cancers to Arthur for this treatment because it provides the highest cure rate and minimizes the risk of recurrences by removing the cancer cells layer by layer until all its roots are gone. It is particularly important to remove skin cancers on the face by this method because the cosmetic results are excellent, whereas cancers removed by the traditional burning, freezing, and other methods can be very disfiguring.

"But what is my face going to look like after you've taken these things off?"

I assured her I would be able to remove her small lesions leaving only faint scars behind. Or, if she wanted, we could try the experimental approach of treating the actinic keratoses with Retin-A, as was being tried in the study.

I knew that the resolution of her medical problem was only the beginning of the help Hillary wanted from me. The second chance she had so plaintively mentioned was her real quest. I scheduled some extra time two weeks after her stitches were removed so we could discuss her need for rejuvenation in light of what I could realistically provide.

We were sitting side by side in front of a mirror. "This is really embarrassing," Hillary said. "To sit here and have someone else seeing exactly what I look at in the mirror—I might as well be naked."

"And I see a striking woman who has accomplished a great deal in her chosen world, who has laughed and smiled and squinted and not cared very well for her skin up until now," I replied. "That's why we're looking in the mirror together. I want to discuss everything we see and what can and can't be changed."

And so, for the next forty minutes, we examined Hillary's face together and planned our attack on those solar stigmata I felt might be amenable to treatment with Retin-A.

I told her that the Retin-A would probably work best on the fine lines around her eyes and some of the thinner vertical rays around her lips. The deeper furrows on either side of her mouth, the lines caused by her smoking, and the thick trench between her eyebrows would, in all probability, need collagen injections to fill them in. Beyond that, more could perhaps be accomplished by a chemical peel. In those days, before liposculpture and laser resurfacing were as refined as they are today, the overall sagging of her skin could only be addressed by a facelift.

"A facelift," she gasped. "Oh no! I'm really against those. Some of my mother's friends have had them, and it's ridiculous. One day they look a haggard seventy, and the next time you see them, they have this tight face that looks like it could break open, perched on top of a turkey-gobbler neck. I'm not trying to make my face lie about my age. I just want to undo whatever damage I can, and I want the change to be subtle, so that David still recognizes me!"

I wanted to level with Hillary about what she could and could not hope for from Retin-A. Although we had seen some remarkable turnarounds in people who had been using it for several years, it usually took many months to have any apparent effect at all. In some cases, Retin-A's effects were hardly noticeable.

Retin-A works in part by increasing the turnover rate of cells in the stratum corneum, the horny outer layer of dead cells that constitutes the epidermal frontier between the internal milieu and the outside world. By early middle age, this process has slowed considerably, leaving a sludge of these dry cells on the face longer. Encouraging the rapid turnover of these dead cells thins the stratum corneum and gives the skin a smoother, rosier look, with a surface that reflects light in a more youthful way. At the same time, the dermis becomes thicker. New blood vessels and new collagen are formed. Fine lines may disappear.

We decided Hillary would begin a regimen of Retin-A three evenings a week, after she had washed her face and let it dry for twenty minutes. In addition, she would wear a hat and sunblock whenever she was outdoors. I would check on her in a month, unless she needed me sooner.

On the subway that evening, as many evenings, I found I had put down the journal I was reading and was instead gazing at the faces surrounding me. Every face was a cipher, registering the sunlight it had been exposed to over the years. Some of the faces, particularly those with darker skin, bore few traces. I noticed an elderly black woman sitting across from me. Her hair was white, and so sparse that her scalp was plainly visible beneath it, but her skin showed none of the "aging" a woman of her age with pale skin and blue or green eyes might have had. Protected from the sun by a heavy mantle of melanin, her face had only the folds and furrows carved there by a lifetime of facial expressions made permanent by the gradual loss of supporting structures and by the relentlessness of gravity. How ironic, I thought, that such hatred has been generated by people's opinions of skin color, when in fact black skin is clearly better adapted to the earthly environment. Black skin *is* beautiful—not only because of its limitless range of shades and colors, but also because of its physiologic perfection. One of my African-American patients once told me that the women she grew up around had a saying about aging: "Good black don't crack." And it's true. While we have many African-American patients, they don't come to us for peels or cosmetic surgery or even skin cancers, for the most part. They simply don't need them.

If Ponce de Leon had ever located the fountain of youth, its waters would, I'm sure, have contained a lot of melanin. Lacking melanin, one can only turn to sun avoidance to stay young-looking. Arthur and I often marvel at Harriet, the African-American woman who cared for Arthur from the day he came home from the hospital as a tiny infant and still, nearly fifty years later, works for his parents as a housekeeper. While the family has aged around her, Harriet's face has developed none of the spots, wrinkles, or skin cancers the others have. All that marks the passage of time are some smile lines around her mouth and eyes and a softening of her jawline and cheeks. From my point of view, this is appropriate aging, the sort we should all strive for.

But, I wondered, could the rate at which faces age have lessons to teach us about the age of the rest of the body? It was around the time I was first treating Hillary King that the concept of biologic age was beginning to emerge as an important topic among researchers. Unlike chronologic age, which reflects the actual number of years since birth, biologic age is an overall representation of the aggregate ages of different organs. Gerontologists at that time were beginning to understand that different organs age at different rates within the same individual. In a study of 1,000 people, begun in 1958 at the Gerontology Research Institute in Baltimore, biologic ages were estimated for various organs according to their level of function. Then a visual estimate was made of each subject's chronologic age. The surprising finding was that on nineteen of twenty-four tests, patients who *looked* older than their true chronologic age also had a higher biologic age. That is to say, their internal organs actually functioned like those of an older person.

But what did all this research mean to a patient like Hillary? What were the connections among time and sun exposure and biologic age? Arthur and other gerontologists are still trying to tease apart all these relationships. There still is no single theory that explains everything we see during the aging process. Almost all of the theories presently being entertained can be grouped into two areas. One camp believes aging is due to cumulative damage to cells from everyday metabolic processes, including oxidative damage caused by free radicals. This theory is supported by the fact that species with a slower basal metabolic rate have a longer life span. Those in the other camp talk about an inborn clock programmed for a certain life span. The observations that different species have different maximum life spans indicate that genetic factors modulate the rate of aging. Additional evidence that genetic determinants are involved comes from studies of human twins; differences in life span are smaller in identical twins than in fraternal twins. By the time I was at Rockefeller, it was clear both groups of theories were important in the understanding of aging.

Environmental and genetic influences are constantly interacting. Several studies have found the degree of skin elasticity to be one of the best markers of biologic age, and one that reflects this interrelationship. Even though skin elasticity normally declines over time, the onset of the decline and the rapidity with which it happens may be partly due to the skin's response to ultraviolet radiation, which in turn is dependent upon a cluster of inherited characteristics. For instance, if the skin responds to the sun with early wrinkling and drooping, this fact may reflect not only the inheritance of less of the protective pigment, melanin, but also the inheritance of less effective enzyme systems for repairing DNA damage, or dysfunction of these systems due to free-radical or other environmental depredations.

In a rare disease called *xeroderma pigmentosum,* these DNA repair systems don't function at all. Patients who have this disorder suffer in a few years the type of light damage that might be anticipated in a Celt farming unprotected from the equatorial sun for many decades. Children with this disease usually develop skin as dry as parchment, dotted with hundreds of frecklelike spots. Their risk of developing skin cancer is at least a thousand times greater than that of the general population. Jeff Potter, a patient of ours with this disease, has a scheduled appointment every Saturday morning at eight o'clock. There are few weeks in the year when there isn't something new to remove from some location on his body. He has had nearly a dozen melanomas in the four years we have been treating him, and countless less serious skin cancers and precancerous moles. Jeff is safer than many with this disease, in that he is under near-constant surveillance by us and by his wife at home. Many people with xeroderma pigmentosum undergo extremely rapid aging, so that by their mid-twenties, they may look like eighty-year-olds. Untreated, these patients die young of their multiple malignancies. I had the mysteries of aging and human life span potential on my mind a great deal in those early days at Rockefeller because of my burgeoning friendship with Arthur Balin. Although I had my own ideas about both matters, it was impossible not to get pulled right into the intense gravitational fields surrounding Arthur. I remember one of our early lunches together in the Rockefeller cafeteria. I sat transfixed as Arthur told me that as far as he was concerned, we had the technology to discover the causes of the aging process, and that whether we could modify this process would depend upon what the actual causes turned out to be. But if animal studies that had already been performed were to be borne out in humans, we should be able to extend the functional human life span.

I was fascinated, of course, by what he said, but philosophically I was influenced by *Gulliver's Travels* and the Struldbruggs, the miserable immortals Gulliver encountered on his odyssey. In fact, soon after that lunch with Arthur I reread that part of Swift's book, which I only dimly remembered from my sophomore year in high school. Swift's clever thought was that even though human beings have always dreamed of immortality, we typically imagine ourselves going on forever with our twenty-year-old minds and bodies. Whereas the unhappy Struldbruggs were stuck in an eternal old age, infirm of body and mind, mocked by the young, and with no hope of a final escape. If we learned to arrest the aging process, I wondered, where would we be able to arrest it, and was it the right thing to do? Wouldn't the planet quickly become overrun, I asked Arthur, if we all lived forever?

"Of course it would," he replied evenly. "That's why humans will have to learn how to colonize space. That's why I'm very interested in biospheres and self-sufficient colonies." As he sat there that afternoon, with the East River rolling behind him, I knew I wanted to work with this man forever. I wanted to be along for the ride as this mind began to flex its muscles.

As much as I wanted to let my thoughts rest on Arthur, my mind returned to Hillary King. I liked her a lot as a patient and as a person, and moreover, I identified with her. Clearly, the devastation of her skin was the result of years of unrelenting environmental punishment. But was she also at the lower end of the spectrum in her ability to clean up the fallout left from bombardment by free radicals? Did the state of her face in fact reflect equal deterioration of some of her internal organs? I hoped not. I hoped her problems lay only skin deep, for that afternoon, in parting, she had shyly mentioned her hope that it wasn't too late to have a baby.

I was actually glad for Hillary that she didn't qualify for the Retin-A study, because of the risk she might have drawn only placebo treatment when clearly we needed to make an aggressive attack on her skin damage. Sister Elizabeth was more ambivalent about healing her damaged skin. During the months we followed her in the study, we watched her face slowly begin to change. She had been instructed to apply the unnamed ointment to her face once or twice a day and then gradually work up to twice-daily applications. In addition, she was to apply a strong sunblock cream every morning to her face and hands.

"My skin certainly feels a lot better," she said one day about a month into the study. "It used to get quite burned after a long day in the sun. It doesn't do that anymore, and it feels much less dry. Maybe this cream will keep it from being so sore this winter too."

The only change we actually recorded at that visit was a slight reconciliation of the two parts of her face. Instead of a sharp line of demarcation where her wimple ended, the skin at the center of her face had begun to fade from its former bronze to a sort of tallowy tan. But although her tan had faded, the formerly unprotected center of her face still bore the lines, liver spots, and freckles of a lifetime in the sun.

We followed Sister Elizabeth for a year. By the end of that year, her face was all one shade, and it was noticeably less dry because of the emollients in the sunscreen she was using, but it was as lined as ever. Certainly no one could have accused Sister Elizabeth of tampering with her age.

"I'm delighted with what you have done," she said at our last appointment. "I must admit, I was a little worried at the beginning that you had some kind of potion that would erase everything familiar on my face. Instead, you've given me very comfortable skin."

When, at the end of the study, we were able to learn which patients had received treatment and which placebo, we found that Sister Elizabeth had indeed received only the placebo. It was the emollient sunscreen that had provided her the skin she wanted—skin that was comfortable and healthy. She developed no more suspicious spots while under the protective cover of the sunblock, and as far as I know, she continues to wear it. I have not seen her since we moved our practice to Pennsylvania.

The decided improvement in Sister Elizabeth's skin exceeded what we would have expected from sun protection alone. But as time has gone on, it has become clear that the use of sunscreen alone does more than just shield the skin. A recent study from Australia showed that among fair-skinned people, not only did those who used a sunscreen with an SPF of 17 develop fewer new precancers than those who used a placebo lotion, but their existing solar keratoses were more likely to go into remission. Other evidence shows that sunscreens actually permit the skin to repair itself somewhat. In some cases, sunscreen alone is even capable of reducing fine lines and improving skin color. Even newer findings suggest that antioxidants, like vitamins A, C, and E, if added to sunscreens, go beyond merely blocking out sunlight and can prevent some of the cell damage and inflammation wrought by UV light. Vitamin E itself has a weak UV blocking effect of its own and, applied topically before sun exposure, can help prevent the initial redness caused by UVB light.

After Hillary had been on the regimen for about two weeks, I got a call that has become familiar over the years I have prescribed Retin-A, particularly in the case of patients who, unlike Sister Elizabeth, were desperate for it to take effect.

"Dr. Pratt," she said, "I didn't know it was going to be like this. I'm not sure this Retin-A is for me."

"What's the matter, Hillary?" I asked, though I had an inkling.

"Well, my skin is just coming off in sheets."

"Hillary, I don't have your chart in front of me. How often are you using the cream?"

"Every night."

"My recollection is that we had talked about your starting out a bit more gradually than that." I was quite sure I had told her to use it three days a week. I almost never advise patients to apply Retin-A more frequently until we see how well they tolerate it. But patients often decide on their own that the prescribed pea-sized amount spread on the face three times a week is too slow in manifesting its reputed magic, so they try double that amount applied daily.

"Some flaking and peeling is normal. It shows the Retin-A is doing its job. The cells of the outer layer of your skin are coming off, and new cells are coming in underneath. The problem is, you're using way too much. I want you to go back to the three-times-per-week level and stay there until your next appointment. Don't forget, also, to let your face dry for at least twenty minutes after you wash it before you apply the Retin-A, and never forget your sunscreen. The new skin that's coming in has no more protection from the sun than a baby's skin."

Over the next six months, Hillary's skin began to make the subtle progress she had hoped for. Her skin became rosier and clearer. Because the dead cells were cycling faster from the surface of her epidermis, light reflected more cleanly off her skin, giving her face a more youthful shine. A few of the spidery-red broken capillaries on her cheeks and nose seemed to disappear as new collagen formed over them. I treated those that remained with an electric needle to coagulate them and cause them to disappear. Eyeing the needle, Hillary began to squirm in her chair. "This looks like it's going to hurt. I want to warn you that even though riders get injured a lot, I don't tolerate pain very well at all."

"We'll start very slowly, and I won't do the ones around your nose until you're used to it. But it's important for you to stay still," I warned. "If it hurts too much, just tell me."

After the first couple of areas, Hillary, who had been sitting as rigid as a child at the dentist's, relaxed. "Oh, that's not bad," she breathed. "I have acupuncture for my back, and it's just like that. Let's do them all!"

The removal of these dilated blood vessels gives an instantaneous improvement to a sun-damaged complexion. Most patients are amazed at the results. The face really does take on a much younger, more feminine appearance after the removal of these chaotic knots of red blood vessels.

I haven't treated Hillary King for the past several years, but she calls occasionally to say hello and order some of the cleansers and moisturizers we have designed. Her husband was sent to work in Germany for several years, and Hillary is busy working with the German coaches who dominate her field of riding. If I were treating her nowadays, when it is clearer that bombardment of genetic material in the cell nucleus by free radicals is a major factor in skin aging, I would urge her to pay attention to her diet. Although good studies are lacking, we are learning, for instance, that a high-fat diet increases the likelihood of developing precancerous spots and perhaps also full-blown skin cancers—again, because such a diet quite possibly increases free-radical formation. Supplemental antioxidants, like beta-carotene and vitamins C and E, can help defend us against these marauding free radicals. Several researchers are exploring the use of topical vitamin C creams whose molecular structure is such that they can penetrate the epidermis and perhaps undo free-radical damage.

Hillary would also be a good candidate for resurfacing using the ultrapulse CO_2 laser. This new technique can take fifteen years off many faces. It removes wrinkles, fine lines, and discolorations while at the same time giving some of the tightening of a facelift.

The last time I saw her, six years after her first appointment, Hillary planned to go on using the Retin-A and SPF 30 sunblock for the rest of her life—as one must to retain its benefits. Although her expression lines still remained and the skin at her jawline was beginning to loosen, the actual texture of her skin was enormously improved. To extend these improvements, I added a mild glycolic acid gel to her cleansing regimen.

"I can't imagine how I'd look by now if I hadn't started this," she said to me when I last saw her. "I'd be a wrinkled old iguana before I was even fifty."

Recently I cut out and added to her file a full-face shot of her from a *Town & Country* story on American horsewomen. It was difficult to tell whether the glow on her face was most due to Retin-A, David, or Granville, her new horse.

Each of these patients, in her own way, showed me there are as many ways of aging as there are people. Whether one chooses to let character develop and register on a face as it will or tries to stabilize the skin at a given point, above all is the human need to feel comfortable in one's own skin. Sister Elizabeth was content being physically comfortable, relieved of the pain of her dry skin. Hillary, on the other hand, reminded me of a line from Lillian Hellman's *Julia:* "There are women who reach a perfect time of life, when the face will never again be as good, the body never as graceful or as powerful." Hillary, like many women, wanted to find her way back in time to that perfect moment. Her body had never failed her, but she wanted her face, once again, to be in concert with it.

The Social Organ

⊙⊙

"We lepers live a long time, and are ironically healthy in other respects. Lusty, though we are loathsome to love. Keen-sighted, though we hate to look upon ourselves. The name of the disease, spiritually speaking, is Humiliation."

JOHN UPDIKE,
"FROM THE JOURNAL OF A LEPER"

It is said that the instinct to avoid those who scratch, who are blemished or scaling, is an impulse programmed into our genes, along with other such survival instincts as fear of fire or revulsion toward tainted meat. Throughout mankind's history, those unfortunates with the characteristic nodules of leprosy, scales of psoriasis, and buboes of plague have been shunned, or worse. Skin diseases, rather than inspiring compassion and nurture, instead are considered repulsive, an expulsion of bodily filth into others' environment. A smooth, healthy skin can be a passport to social success. Publicus Syrius, in 42 B.C., wrote, "A fair exterior is a silent recommendation." The blemished may be excommunicated.

Leprosy, a bacterial disease, is perhaps the prototype in the collective mind for all socially ruinous skin diseases. Leviticus 13 in the Old Testament is a veritable treatise on dermatologic diagnostic criteria and treatment algorithms for what is referred to as *leprosy* in most translations but that medical historians now tell us probably encompassed a wide range of skin eruptions. It is likely that those unfortunates with psoriasis, vitiligo, perhaps even severe acne or ringworm, received the leper's treatment. Throughout history, diseases of the skin have caused a degree of social anguish on a par only with diseases of the mind. Compassion could hardly be considered the order of the day when we learn from Leviticus 13:45–46,

> The leper who has the disease shall wear torn clothes
> and let the hair of his head hang loose, and he shall cover
> his upper lip and cry, "Unclean, unclean."
> He shall remain unclean as long as he has the disease;
> he is unclean; he shall dwell alone in a habitation outside
> the camp.

I once had a patient whose skin condition, while neither unusual nor extreme in itself, was for her, because of ancient fears and ignorance, a threat to all she held dear in life.

Chandrika Das was only twenty-five the first time she came to our office. She was my last patient of the day one dreary November afternoon. When I opened the door to my examination room, where she was waiting, I was surprised to see a short Indian woman in a bright apple-green sari embroidered with gold. She seemed to light up the entire room.

"Good afternoon, Mrs. Das," I said, shaking her hand. I smiled at her, but she didn't smile back. In fact, the dampness around her eyes suggested she had recently been weeping. "How can I help you today?"

"I am desperately in need of your help, Dr. Pratt," she said in a formal but singsong British accent. "I am developing white spots on my body. I am afraid it might be leprosy."

Leprosy, or Hansen's disease, is caused by *Mycobacterium leprae*, a bacterium in the same family as those that cause tuberculosis. Although we tend to think of leprosy as a biblical scourge or a disease of the deepest tropics, there are actually more than ten million cases in the world today—particularly in Asia and Africa, but also in the United States, among immigrants from the Third World. Contrary to the dreadful images many of us carry in our minds of colonies of pitiful creatures with rotting flesh and missing limbs, leprosy may appear only as white plaques, rashes, and nodules, although people with the more severe forms may suffer nerve damage, blindness, hair loss, and deformities. In darker-skinned races, leprosy may first show up as lighter patches of skin, which later thicken and turn white.

"I will want to examine your skin, and then you can point out to me the areas you're concerned about, but first I need to know a bit more about you," I said. After we had discussed Chandrika's general health and medical and personal history, I asked her to go into the examining room and change into a gown.

While she was changing, I reviewed my notes. Chandrika was married to a man who was attending the Wharton School of Economics at the University of Pennsylvania. They had lived in Philadelphia for a year and were planning to return to India after her husband, Raj, had finished his studies at Wharton. Chandrika herself worked part-time in the library.

Chandrika's skin was a pleasure to behold. It was smooth and undamaged, the color of butterscotch. There were virtually no moles or other lesions the length of her body, except for a white patch on the inside of each wrist and a small pale area at the corner of her right eye.

"Are these the areas you're concerned about?" I asked her.

"Yes," she said, holding up her wrists. "So far I have been very lucky, because the spots are small, and I have been able to keep them hidden from my husband."

"Why?" I asked her, surprised. "Why do you worry about hiding them from your husband?"

"In India, people with white spots have very bad problems, because many people think they have leprosy. My husband would not have married me if he had known I have this disease. There is no way my father could have paid a big enough dowry."

The patches she showed me had jagged edges and looked chalk-white against the uniform tan of her skin. I couldn't be positive what they were until I had examined them under the black light dermatologists call a Wood's light. A Wood's light is useful for determining both the extent of pigmentary abnormalities and the level of the skin at which they are occurring. As I got the Wood's lamp out, I asked her again about hiding her lesions from her husband.

"What would your husband do if he knew you had these spots?"

"I don't know what he *would* do, Dr. Pratt. But what he *could* do is divorce me. That would be his right."

"On what grounds?" I was fascinated and horrified.

"On the grounds that I am diseased, imperfect, unclean, and that I might pass this on to our children."

Under the Wood's lamp, with the room lights turned off, Chandrika's lesions stood out white as moonlight. This meant they were completely depigmented, with no melanin to absorb the light. This in itself was fairly conclusive evidence that she had *vitiligo*, a common skin disease that afflicts about one percent of the population worldwide. A number of other diseases cause a decrease in normal pigmentation, but each has distinguishing features not evident on Chandrika's skin. One of the most common causes of white spots on the skin is the condition *tinea versicolor*, caused by a fungus. But under the Wood's light, the apparently white spots of tinea would show up tan rather than white, because they are not completely depigmented. Moreover, the lesions tend to be scaly, while those of vitiligo are not, and tinea is more common on the chest, neck, back, and upper arms.

"Mrs. Das, I think you have a disease called vitiligo. You definitely don't have any form of leprosy. Vitiligo is not at all uncommon, and it can be treated. But I will need to take a small sample of your skin to send to the lab so that I can be absolutely certain."

"Can you stop it before it spreads? I have seen people in India whose entire skin is covered with these white patches. If they are women, they often suffer a great deal. So far, I have been lucky. I have been able to hide my disease, but every day I lock myself in the bathroom, and I check to see if there is more. I am so worried. I can't expect you to understand. You are an educated woman from a country where men and women are equal. But I hope you can help me."

It had been many years since gender had been much of an issue in my life. My mind struggled with the implications of what Chandrika was saying. The very thought that a man did not necessarily agree to marry a woman in sickness and in health was still shocking to my Western view, even though I knew it was the way in so many countries. The closest I had come before to such a situation was when a young patient begged me to remove a small heart-shaped tattoo she had on her shoulder, because she was marrying into a Greek family in whose culture only prostitutes or gypsies had tattoos.

"I'm so surprised at what you're telling me," I said to Chandrika. "I thought so much had changed in India. What about Indira Gandhi? What about all the Indian women who are doctors?" I checked myself. I wanted to be empathic and certainly not appear disparaging of her country, but I found myself indignant that such brutality could be countenanced just because a woman had a common skin disease, one that wasn't even contagious. To me, it seemed akin to a man's having the right to divorce his wife simply because she was ugly.

"You are quite right, Dr. Pratt. Much has changed in India, but much has stayed the same. What is law and what is done in the privacy of the family are often quite different. A woman with a skin disease like this is nearly unmarriageable unless she has a very large dowry. Even men may have difficulty getting jobs if people can see that they have white spots on their skin. My husband is an educated man, but he comes from a traditional family, and in India, the family is very powerful. My grandmother had white leprosy, and she was cast out of her husband's family. She was fortunate, because her own family took her back. That is why I am so frightened. Could I have inherited this, and will it get worse?"

"Sometimes it is inherited, but not always. As for its course, vitiligo can be hard to predict. Sometimes it stays the same for a long time and then progresses slowly or very rapidly. Occasionally some of the white areas darken again on their own, although not usually to the same degree as the rest of the skin."

"So you are saying that I may not be able to keep this a secret."

"I'm saying I can't promise you that you won't get more spots. There are ways of helping those you do have disappear, but it may take a year or more before the lighter areas will match the rest of your skin, and you may need to come to the office for treatment as often as twice a week. Also, I cannot guarantee that the treatment will work for you. Since you have such a small area that is affected, you might actually prefer to use a camouflage makeup or a self-tanning product and wait to see whether the disease spreads. At the same time, I will give you a steroid cream that you can apply to the spots. It isn't as effective as some of the other treatments, but it's worth a try, because your vitiligo is very localized."

"What is it that causes this disease?" she asked.

"The cause of vitiligo is unknown," I told her, "although there are several theories." One suggests it may be the result of an autoimmune process in which the patient's immune system fails to distinguish between the patient's own melanin-producing cells and foreign invaders like viruses. Vitiligo patients often carry in their blood antibodies to their own pigment cells, showing that the immune system has at some point read them as foreign. Vitiligo often shows up in patients who have other autoimmune problems, so we always draw blood to test them for serious internal diseases that may have been flagged for us by the skin spots.

Patients with both the deadly skin cancer, melanoma, and vitiligo have antibodies against similar antigens that are present on both melanocytes (melanin-producing cells) and melanomas, which are essentially cancerous melanocytes. What happens to people with vitiligo—the selective destruction of their melanocytes—is actually the goal of melanoma therapy. There's some suggestion that patients with melanomas who later develop vitiligo actually have a better prognosis than usual, which again suggests a link between them.

Another current theory of vitiligo is that some abnormal nervous system chemical may destroy melanocytes or otherwise suppress melanin production. This theory is based on the fact that vitiligo occasionally develops in patients who have undergone nerve injury, as well as in psychiatric patients and those suffering from emotional stress. It is also supported by animal studies that may not be readily generalizable to humans. For instance, rats may lose pigmentation when injected with adrenaline, and electrical stimulation of skin nerves can cause loss of pigmentation in fish.

The third theory suggests that some toxic product may be released during melanin synthesis and that normal melanocytes have built-in protection against these toxins. The failure of this protective system, it is suggested, could result in vitiligo.

"All right," Chandrika sighed after listening attentively. "I guess I'll just have to try the things you give me to use at home and pray that they help."

"Since you have been covering your vitiligo, I want to give you some cream that ought to work better, in that it won't rub off or wash off. We can match it to your exact skin shade."

I was confident by then of my ability to match a patient's skin color closely without a lot of trial and error. It hadn't always been so. One of my most humiliating adolescent memories concerns my clumsy efforts at making myself attractive to my high school gym teacher. After poring over each issue of *Seventeen* magazine, I was convinced I needed to wear more makeup. I decided a generous rub of blusher on either cheek would make me look far more attractive. After carefully applying enough to give myself what I perceived, in the fluorescent light of the school bathroom, to be a healthy glow, I joined the rest of the class.

Several sets of eyes seemed to linger on my face an unaccustomedly long time, but far and away the greatest number of stares were bestowed by the object of my wiles, Mr. Lutz himself. After class, he made a beeline for me. Suddenly I found my face throbbing from an entirely natural blush. The makeup was working better than I could have dared hope! All of a sudden I wasn't quite certain how to behave and was just trying to figure that out when Mr. Lutz took me by the elbow and marched me out of the room.

"I'm going to call your mother so she can come get you. Your face is so red, you must have a high fever. I think you should stay away from the other students until she arrives."

By the time I began mixing concealers and foundations for my patients, my skills had decidedly improved. After a few minutes of mixing, I came up with a good match for Chandrika. I applied a light covering over the spots and blended it into the surrounding skin.

"Here, take a look," I said, handing her a mirror.

"But that's wonderful!" she cried. "I've never been able to buy makeup in this country. I should have come to you instead of going to Wanamaker's."

"At least you won't have to worry about this coming off."

"Well, that's certainly an improvement," she said with a rueful smile.

I also gave her a prescription for a moderately potent steroid cream that might possibly take care of her spots and told her I'd be in touch in a couple of days. She asked me not to call her at home with the biopsy and blood test results but, rather, to leave word at the university library where she worked. She made an appointment to come back in to have the stitches removed from the biopsy site on her wrist and to let me check her progress with the topical steroid therapy.

After her sutures were removed, Chandrika did not come in again for several months. She called to tell me she didn't think the steroid cream was making any difference and that she had stopped using it. She said she was happy with the camouflage makeup and was going to hope no new spots would appear.

Nearly a year later, again in the late autumn, I got a message that Chandrika had called and seemed very upset. When I reached her at the library, her voice sounded panicked. "The spots are starting to grow," she said. "Two weeks ago, I noticed a few little white freckles near the spots on my wrists. Now I have more, and they seem to be spreading up my arm. There is a big spot near the inside of my left elbow, and I think I am beginning to get it around my mouth. Please, Dr. Pratt, please help me! I know your schedule is booked tight and that you are very busy, but please see me as soon as possible. This is just what I was afraid of."

When Chandrika came in, it was clear her disease was reactivating. There was no way to tell what its course would be. In extreme cases, vitiligo can depigment virtually the entire body over the course of several weeks. Clearly, Chandrika needed immediate treatment and not just makeup.

"Chandrika, I don't want to frighten you, but I think you need additional treatment. I want you to keep using the cream, because it is actually now when the disease is rapidly spreading that these creams can help the most. But I also think it's time for you to start light therapy. It is usually effective, but as I told you, it requires frequent visits to the office, where we give you a medication that makes your skin more sensitive to light and then expose you to ultraviolet light. The problem is that you just won't be able to hide what you're doing. You have to wear sunglasses for twenty-four hours after each treatment, and your skin may become less easy to camouflage, because the treatment often temporarily causes the healthy skin to darken."

"But what am I going to do?" she cried. "I feel as if I have nowhere to hide, and I don't know what will happen if my husband finds out."

I noticed her small hands were trembling and twisting in her lap. "Chandrika, I have a suggestion. I think you should bring your husband into the office to discuss the situation. If you feel that he would be more comfortable talking to another man, he could meet with my husband, Dr. Balin, whose office is upstairs. The point is, you need treatment. This is a common skin disease that has nothing to do with leprosy. It's not contagious. Dr. Balin or I could explain this to your husband. He is an educated man. I am certain we can make him understand."

She shook her head. "I don't know which is worse—to try to keep hiding or to risk having him get angry or even leave me."

"Chandrika, I have to be very honest. It's entirely possible you will not be able to hide the problem much longer. Wouldn't it be better to be honest with your husband and stop living with this uncertainty?"

She sighed deeply and withdrew her hand. Then she looked off into space for a moment. "All right, I know you are right. I know you are busy, but is there any way you could call him in the morning and see him tomorrow? That way I will be at work, and I won't have to try to explain why you want to see him."

"Of course I can. I'll make time."

When I reached Raj Das by telephone the next morning, he sounded impatient and confused. "But Chandrika mentioned nothing to me. It can't be terribly serious. Why can't we discuss this matter over the telephone, Doctor?" he asked. "I am trying to study, and I have very little time."

But I was firm that I wanted to meet in person, and he agreed to come later that afternoon. Putting down the telephone, I hoped I wasn't going to embroil myself in a familial and perhaps cultural situation I didn't fully understand, but it seemed the only way to make Chandrika's situation better.

The man who was shown into my office was quite different from what I had expected. His rather abrupt manner on the telephone that morning had led me to wonder whether Chandrika was perhaps correct in thinking he might not take the news well. But standing before me was a man with a kind, intelligent face. His limpid black eyes were worried, not at all suspicious. I couldn't imagine this man turning on his wife.

"Mr. Das," I began, "Chandrika has a skin disease, and it needs to be treated. She was worried about your reaction, so I told her I would discuss the situation with you personally, face to face."

"Is Chandrika ill?"

"Your wife has a skin disease called vitiligo, which can make areas of the skin lose their normal coloration. It is treatable, and it is not contagious. I wanted you to come in because I wanted to reassure you and answer in person any questions you might have."

"Vitiligo!" he said, his face flooding with relief. "I know what vitiligo is. A friend of mine at university had vitiligo. Why then, Chandrika is in no danger. I have been frightened all day, wondering what might be the matter. I tried to call her at work but have been unable to reach her. As you say, vitiligo can be treated. The chap I knew came to look like one of those spotted horses before he went to the doctor, but now he is completely recovered. Can't my wife be treated the same way?"

"Yes, Mr. Das, she can. I will tell her you understand the need for her to begin treatment, and we can get her started right away."

"Quite a tempest in a teapot," he said, shaking his head. "I am surprised Chandrika didn't mention any of this to me. She is a beautiful girl. I would hate for her to delay her treatment. But . . . I have noticed no vitiligo on my wife. Are you sure?"

I wasn't certain how to be politic. I didn't necessarily want to tell him his wife had been hiding her condition from him for many months. "Your wife has only a very few light spots, which she has been keeping covered with makeup, because she was worried you would find her disease offensive."

"What a silly girl. I thought she knew me better than that."

"She said that in India vitiligo is often confused with leprosy."

"Yes, by ignorant people perhaps. I remember my friend was worried people would think he had leprosy, and now that you mention it, he too tried just to cover up his white spots. We used to laugh at him for wearing makeup. My poor wife," he said again, shaking his head as he rose to leave.

Chandrika came in to see me a few days later, looking more relaxed than at either of her other appointments. "Dr. Pratt, thank you for having the good sense to stop me from trying to hide," she said. "I realize now Raj would have been more upset that I was keeping the truth from him."

I planned to treat Chandrika using phototherapy, a type of

treatment that probably had its origins in her own country and ancient Egypt. Folk remedies for treating "leprosy" involved the use of several plant extracts. The plants referred to in ancient medical texts were probably some of the many that contain psoralens, a class of chemicals that react with ultraviolet light and stimulate pigment formation. When I think about the earliest healers who chose these plants from among the hundreds at their disposal, I am amazed by their sophistication. What could have led them to exactly the right plants? So many of our most effective pharmaceuticals are derived from purified plant extracts: Valium from valerian root; vincristine, an anticancer drug, from vinca, the ground cover known as myrtle. Reserpine, a blood-pressure drug, comes from Cimcifuga, or the shady border plant snakeroot; digitalis, for heart failure, comes from foxglove. There are so many. One wonders whether humans have an innate ability to identify plants with healing properties.

At the turn of the century, vitiligo was treated with topical application of psoralens followed by exposure to sunlight. Nowadays, we usually prefer to treat patients with topical or oral psoralens and controlled exposures to ultraviolet A light, which penetrates deep into the skin. In many cases, this combination (known as PUVA) will result in complete repigmentation. Areas that have been fully repigmented usually do not relapse, although other areas of the body may develop new spots of vitiligo and the disease may continue to progress.

Dark-skinned individuals who have vitiligo over more than half their bodies are usually better treated by depigmentation—completely bleaching their skin—rather than attempting repigmentation using PUVA. This is an extreme treatment, using a drug called monobenzylether of hydroquinone. Although not everyone can tolerate this treatment, those who can permanently lose all their pigment and become very light-skinned.

Chandrika was eager to get started with the PUVA therapy. I explained she would need to come in to be treated twice a week to start and that we might increase her treatments to three sessions per week, depending upon how she tolerated the PUVA. Maximal repigmentation was likely to take a year or more, and it was important that she not become pregnant during that time, because of possible damage to a developing fetus. She would need to wear a sunblock and as much clothing as she could to protect her skin totally from the sun. Uncontrolled exposure to sun is, of course, extra dangerous for patients taking light-sensitizing psoralens, which are like anti-sunblocks. Psoralens are also taken up by the lenses of the eyes, which become more sensitive to ultraviolet light and therefore more prone to developing cataracts. We tell our patients to wear sunglasses outdoors for the first twenty-four hours after each treatment.

Chandrika tolerated the therapy well, with little of the redness and scaling some patients develop after exposure to the lights. After about four months, we began to see some response, particularly in the newer spots on her arms and chest. The returning pigment cells first come up through the hair follicles, forming dark pinpoints in the blanched areas. Gradually these pinpoints enlarge to polka dots, which coalesce. The normal skin, which is also reacting to the PUVA, becomes temporarily darker. After a year, the spots all the way up to Chandrika's elbows had melded with the rest of her skin, but the small areas around her eye and mouth had not responded completely, which meant they had a higher likelihood of enlarging.

One day, Chandrika asked the nurse if she could speak to me after her light treatment. When I came in to see her, she said, "Dr. Pratt, please do not think I am ungrateful for all the help you have given me. You have helped me so much I don't know how to thank you enough, but I think this will be my last treatment, at least for a while. Raj and I have decided we just don't want to wait any longer before starting a family. I don't mind using makeup on these few remaining areas. You have done such an excellent job with the rest of my skin, and I now know that the disease can be controlled somewhat."

I bade Chandrika good-bye and good luck. About a year and a half later, she sent me a photograph of their baby daughter, Madhavi. Raj got a teaching appointment at Stanford, and the family had decided to remain in America for several more years. Last year, Chandrika's Christmas card, which now showed a family of three children, mentioned that her vitiligo had returned. She had found an Indian dermatologist in San Francisco and was once again receiving PUVA therapy.

I sometimes think about how the story would have turned out if

Raj had been other than the understanding, enlightened man he was. While at first I felt certain that Chandrika must be overreacting, perhaps on the basis of what had happened to her grandmother, I later met an Indian immunologist at a dermatology meeting Arthur and I attended. "She had every right to be nervous, the poor girl," this woman told me. "Perhaps especially in educated families, vitiligo and other diseases that resemble leprosy are extremely stigmatizing. I think it is something deep within the Indian psyche, left over from the days when leprosy was a greater threat. Many in India would still consider such a woman untouchable in all senses of the word."

I find the word "untouchable" a chilling one. The AIDS epidemic has created a new class of untouchables. Men and women who carry the most common cutaneous emblem of the disease, the telltale purple lesions of Kaposi's sarcoma, are made all the more miserable by their constant awareness of the abhorrence they inspire. And, as in the time of Leviticus, plenty of "leaders" would excommunicate these contemporary "unclean" through various draconian measures ranging from quarantine to branding.

As a doctor with two young children, I am as frightened of AIDS as anyone else. I was just starting med school when the first cases of GRID (gay-related immunodeficiency disease), as it was then called, were appearing. Many of the doctors around me remained quite cavalier about their own infection risk from this pathogen, which seemed, at the time, to be the more or less exclusive province of sexually active gay men. But I began to wear gloves pretty much every time I examined a patient. As it has turned out, this was a good habit to have developed for the assurance of my own safety. So much is unknown about HIV. While it is clear that non-sexually-acquired cases rely on transmission through blood, it is still theoretically possible the virus may be transmitted by other routes—including the shedding of langerhans cells, which are immune cells in the epidermis known to carry the virus. If this has happened, it hasn't yet been described in the literature. But I am a mother first, and I recognize that my own occupation does carry risks to my family. I must pay attention even to theoretical routes of transmission. Wearing gloves and, when needed, a mask and glasses makes me feel less vulnerable. Even so, my mind is divided on the issue of latex examination gloves. Everything I know in my heart about healing underscores the importance of touch and the rich universe of nonverbal messages it can convey. It makes me sad that I have to draw such a firm boundary between my patients and myself. Sometimes I can't do it.

During my internal medicine residency, I spent quite a lot of time taking care of the legions of HIV-infected patients beginning to inundate the New York City hospitals. I'll never forget something that happened with one of my patients, a young man named Harrison, who was back in the hospital with only a few days to live. By this point in his illness, he was totally blind from the invasion of his eyes by cytomegalovirus, one of the hordes of bugs that seize the easy opportunity of colonizing a patient whose immune system can't fight back. As I was taking off my examination gloves and preparing to drop them into the wastebasket, Harrison suddenly spoke up.

"Dr. Pratt," he said. "Put your gloves back on."

"Why?" I asked, confused.

"Because I want to hold your hand."

I did not put my gloves back on. Who could have? In recalling that farewell handclasp with Harrison, I ask myself how I would react today, and my thoughts are divided. The physician and mother in me warn me to look out for myself and my children first, so that one breach of the infection barrier doesn't make me unable to be a mother or to practice medicine. On the other hand, the healer in me is ashamed at the edicts of the pragmatic parent and physician who feels she is witholding from patients who need it most that extra dimension of medicine—healing hands.

Arthur is much less worried than I am. This is in part because he spent many more years than I in the pre-AIDS medical world, where one rarely wore latex gloves outside the operating room.

"Why should I put on my gloves to examine a grandmother who's been married for fifty years?" he'll say.

"But how do you know she didn't have surgery a year ago with massive blood transfusions?" I'll reply. "Just do it for the sake of the children. We still don't know all there is to know about the transmission of this virus."

•   •   •

Jonathan Harris came from a culture where there was little superstition or outright ignorance concerning his common skin disease. He had none of Chandrika's problems, and his skin disease was a household word and not threatening to anyone else. Nevertheless, Jonathan had spent most of his life trying not to be distressed by others' reactions to his severe psoriasis, and he was tiring of the battle.

Jonathan brought two pictures with him on his first visit. One, from the *Hartford Courant* in November 1947, showed him in a Yale football uniform following that year's Harvard-Yale game. The other, taken a year later, showed Jonathan in the dhoti-like garment sometimes worn by subjects in older medical photographs, with a black bar printed across his eyes. This photograph, he told me, was taken from a paper on psoriasis that had appeared in *Archives of Dermatology* sometime in 1948.

"It looks like you had a pretty bad case," I said. "When did you first get it?"

"I was about eight or nine when I first recall developing a little patch, but as far as I can remember, it wasn't diagnosed at that time. It was just a red patch that bothered me a lot, because it was right where my glasses rubbed."

It wasn't until Jonathan started playing football in high school that his psoriasis began to spread. It began with two scaly red patches, one on the back of each hand. (This symmetry is typical of psoriasis and sometimes occurs to a remarkable degree. One often sees patients whose lesions are distributed almost like two halves of an inkblot.) These were soon followed by more plaques on his arms, face, ears, and even on his scalp.

"It was a bad time to get a skin disease," Jonathan said. "Everyone was used to kids with bad acne, even though they weren't always very nice to them, but what I had on my chest and hands made me almost a leper. Except for my small circle of friends, I was ostracized. My nickname was 'Flako.' I pretended to laugh along with them, but inside I was terribly humiliated. I used to wish I could get psoriasis anywhere but on the face I had to show the world. I remember we once had a movie in science class, and it was all about skin diseases. People kept turning around and looking at me and whispering. I thought I'd die of self-consciousness."

Finally, Jonathan's family doctor had recommended a camouflage called "Lydia O'Leary's Covermark," which helped hide the red patches on his face. "It really did wonders for my appearance—and my self-respect," he said. "At least I was able to get an occasional date."

While at Yale, his psoriasis remained in a steady state, but Jonathan sought out a dermatologist to see whether he could actually rid him of the disease. "First he tried injections of arsenic, but they didn't work. Then he tried coal tar, which helped a little. Finally, he gave me some ointment that looked like Vaseline, but it helped loosen the hard plaques. That treatment left me with red blotches, but they were better than the flaking elephant skin I had before. By my last year at Yale, I was in pretty good shape."

To someone who hasn't seen firsthand a skin ravaged by psoriasis, it is difficult to understand how devastating it can be. When most people think of psoriasis, they think of a flaking scalp and television advertisements for over-the-counter psoriasis treatment. But psoriasis can be so invasive and difficult to control that it can make life truly miserable. In all the scientific literature, there is probably no better account of the nature of the disease than in this description in the essay "From the Diary of a Leper," by John Updike, who has been afflicted with severe and extensive psoriasis since childhood:

> The form of the disease is as follows: spots, plaques and avalanches of excess skin, manufactured by the dermis through some trifling but persistent error in its metabolic instructions, expand and slowly migrate across the body like lichen on a tombstone. I am silvery, scaly. Puddles of flakes form wherever I rest my flesh. Each morning, I vacuum my bed.

There are actually several types of psoriasis, but the underlying problem in all of them is overproduction of epidermal cells. Instead of adhering to the twenty-one- to twenty-eight-day cycle that normally governs the turnover of epidermal cells, those afflicted with psoriasis race through this cycle in three or four days. Instead of shedding normally and being replaced, these cells build up on the skin and cause it to thicken and crack or scale. At the same time, new, immature cells keep pushing up from beneath, creating a cutaneous logjam where epidermal cells pile up on one another. The epidermis may grow to five to ten times its normal thickness. New blood vessels are formed to bring blood to the lesions, which causes the plaques to look red and inflamed. Picking at the scales makes them bleed easily.

Psoriasis is quite a common affliction. About 2 percent of the population is affected to some degree. Although psoriasis may be so mild it goes unrecognized, it generally shows up as red patches underlying tough, scaly plaques that resemble the horny growths called "chestnuts" on the inside of horses' legs. Psoriasis most often affects the elbows, knees, scalp, back, and buttocks, although in the worst cases, it is everywhere. About half of all patients with psoriasis have pitting and discoloration of their fingernails, a manifestation that can be maddeningly difficult to treat. Psoriasis is often associated with one type of arthritis, although the connection between the two is not well understood.

Just after he left Yale and returned to Massachusetts to take over his father's printing business, Jonathan experienced his worst flare-up. "I had it everywhere, and I mean *everywhere*," he said with a laugh. "Of course, the timing was about as bad as it could be. I was getting married in December, and here it was June. Thank God my wife-to-be stuck by me. Her parents were convinced I had syphilis!"

Jonathan was admitted to Massachusetts General. It was here that he was photographed for the journal.

"I had one of the worst cases the doctors there had ever seen. They kept me for about a month. I had salt baths every day to loosen the plaques, and they covered me with coal tar ointment and put me under lights twice a day. I was quite a sight. They made us wear the same tar-caked robes twenty-four hours a day. I remember the doctors used to tell us that they knew they were using enough tar if our robes stood up by themselves! I felt like I had been tarred and feathered, but it worked."

This type of intensive, in-hospital treatment of psoriasis patients used to be more common. In earlier times, patients would often plan their vacations from work so they could check into the hospital for a month. After about a month their psoriasis would clear, often not to return for a year. Although Arthur and I have several patients at the moment who would probably respond to this type of regimen, it's almost impossible in the era of health care "reform." No matter the superior efficacy, insurers will not pay for hospital treatments they feel can be done on an outpatient basis.

Over the years, numerous treatment regimens have been developed to control psoriasis. Coal tar has been used for over a century. It probably works by slowing the exuberant epidermal overgrowth characteristic of the disease. However, there are thousands of chemicals in crude tar, and no one has been able to separate and catalog them all, so we don't have any idea which of them are actually active against psoriasis. Nowadays, purified tars in cosmetic bases are available, but alas, they don't work as well as the crude tars in all their stickiness and malodorousness.

A later variant was a synthetic coal tar derivative called *anthralin*. This medication, like coal tar, is still in use today, particularly in England, where it is considered a mainstay of treatment. Nowadays, however, coal-derived preparations come in gel, stick, and ointment forms. While they still stain clothes and have a distinctive odor, they are a far cry from the cruder medications of the early part of the century. In 1925, a variation known as the *Goeckerman regimen* was introduced by a dermatologist at the Mayo Clinic. The psoriasis scales are first painted with the tar. After a couple of hours, the tar is partially removed and the area bathed with ultraviolet B light, which boosts the action of the tar. Patients with extensive plaques can be treated in an enclosed cabinet that exposes their entire body to the light. Often a few months of this treatment is enough to make the psoriasis go away for six months or even a year. Patients with severe psoriasis may need to be treated daily just to keep their disease in check.

"I've got to hand it to them, they did make me presentable for my wedding," Jonathan continued. "In fact, I was almost completely clear."

Five years later, Jonathan decided to expand the family business. He and his wife would move to Philadelphia, where Jonathan would open a new office.

"At that point, I was in good shape. I still had a few patches on my scalp and my elbows, but they stayed pretty stable. Then, all of a sudden, I started to have flare-ups again. Looking back on it, I think it was stress-related. We were new parents, I was working round the clock trying to get the branch office up and running. It was an exhausting time, with a lot of uncertainty."

Indeed, there is evidence that psoriasis may be made worse by emotional stress, particularly in children. I remember a truck driver Arthur treated for many years. He had only two small patches of psoriasis on his elbows that never spread. One night, driving along a slick highway in his eighteen-wheeler, he collided with a VW beetle, killing the seventeen-year-old driver. Two days later, psoriasis erupted all over his body.

Trauma to the skin, in the form of cuts, abrasions, or even severe sunburn or chafing shoes or clothes, can also trigger psoriasis. People with psoriasis often find they develop new areas of psoriasis at the site of skin trauma. This is called the *Koebner phenomenon,* or "koebnerization."

"I hadn't been self-conscious about my problem for years," Jonathan said. "I guess that was thanks to my loving, loyal wife, who seemed not even to notice that everywhere I went, I left scales—in the tub, in the bed, in my clothes. But to suddenly turn into the Elephant Man at a time when I was supposed to be talking to prospective clients was really, really tough. If they don't have anything wrong with their appearance, there's no way most people can appreciate what it's like to be the subject of furtive glances, double takes, what it's like to have people give a funny little wave instead of shaking your hand, to have store clerks drop your change on the counter rather than hand it to you. Suddenly, I found myself on very shaky ground. All the self-confidence you need to start up a business was shot. I was scared I wasn't going to be able to pull it off, and the more I worried, the more I flared. And the more I flared, the more alarming my appearance became!"

At this point, the psoriasis was so severe that just moving was enough to make Jonathan's affected skin crack into deep, painful fissures. That was in 1959. At his wife's urging, he located a dermatologist in Philadelphia who would treat him with the coal tar and ultraviolet light therapy that had helped him in the past. Many psoriasis patients are helped by UV light, even without tars. In fact, many patients, John Updike among them, find sunbathing a highly effective way of keeping their disease in check. Most doctors prefer controlled UV exposures in the office, because a severe sunburn can koebnerize psoriasis. However, this time, the exposure was less than well controlled. After positioning Jonathan in the light box, the doctor turned on the timer and left to check on another patient.

"Well I sat there, and I sat there, waiting for him to come back or the timer to turn the lights off. My skin started to get very hot and red. I realized I was burning. I finally just got up and walked out into the hallway. I was cherry red and scalding hot all over. I never went back to that doctor, and after that, I really didn't want to be treated with lights—ever."

In desperation, Jonathan went to his family doctor, who prescribed two topical steroids. After applying the creams, Jonathan was to cover the areas with a thick coat of Vaseline. This is a treatment still in use today, and it worked well for Jonathan for a number of years. He continued to have flare-ups, and every time he cut or scraped himself he developed another spot of psoriasis in the wound, but the disease seemed to be in check.

"For a while, it cleared up almost completely," he told me. "I still had it on my back and on my hands, but it was nothing like what it had been. I can't say my skin looked completely normal, because where there had been psoriasis, I got little white spots, kind of like freckles in reverse."

Even though his skin was fairly clear for a number of years, life with psoriasis was never completely normal. "I always felt like I was on borrowed time, because by then I knew how bad it could be and that it could come back any time. It affected my life in all kinds of ways. Unlike lots of people with psoriasis, the sun didn't help me one bit. This was before they had sunblocks and all that, so what I really had to do was stay out of the sun. I always wore long sleeves, both to keep the sun out and to hide the psoriasis. I remember one day telling my ten-year-old daughter that she'd have to wait for her mom to come home to take her to the lake and she said to me, 'What's the matter, Dad? Are you embarassed to go swimming with your fish scales?' That hurt, but children don't know. Even my wife was afraid that Katie might have inherited psoriasis."

Jonathan came to our office in 1994. Although he had been experiencing alternate flaring and clearing of his skin for over twenty years, he was in the middle of one of the worst flare-ups of his life, he told me that day. There had been some difficult changes in his life. In the previous year, his adored wife of nearly forty years had died of cancer, and his children were grown and scattered across the country. He wasn't ready to withdraw from life yet. "I like being married," he confided. "I've been married most of my life, and it agrees with me, but where do you find a woman who's willing to put up with a man whose skin flakes off?" He gave a little laugh. "I've been passing your sign for years, but I always figured you and your husband would be like the rest of the doctors I've seen over the years, who couldn't really do much for me. Up until recently the creams have been working fairly well, but I've got it bad now."

He was quite accurate in his claim of having psoriasis "everywhere." Large, scaly plaques covered his back and chest, he had large patches on the back of each hand extending up to his elbows, and his feet and lower legs were similarly afflicted. Besides the psoriasis, he had a probable skin cancer on the tip of his nose, as well as several more suspicious lesions on his scalp and on the tips of his ears. I explained the biopsy procedure to him and then got to work.

Arthur recently asked me to come in while he talked to a woman with another type of severe psoriasis, of a type called *pustular psoriasis.* This is a much rarer form of the disease, generally limited to the palms and soles. People with pustular psoriasis develop groups of yellowish pustules that form rapidly and soon flatten and turn dark brown. They may scale, or deep, painful fissures may develop in the involved skin. In Bonnie Williams's case, the disease had appeared in middle age. Prior to the first outbreak, she had been conscious for several years of a flaking red spot on the side of each foot. Even before they appeared, she had had a red spot that resembled a burn on the back of one of her hands for many years, but although she had never been able to make it go away, she had never worried about it. It wasn't until she went for a pedicure and the pedicurist attempted to shave off two calluses on her heels that her psoriasis erupted.

"From there it just took off like wildfire," she told Arthur. "It went all the way around my feet and onto the soles." Soon her feet were so painful, she could barely walk. The spots on her hands gradually enlarged, until the two dime-sized spots were the size of quarters. Other psoriatic lesions developed on her palms.

"You have no idea how impossible my life has become," she said. "I've heard people joke about 'the heartbreak of psoriasis,' but it's no joke. I've lived alone ever since my husband died, and all of a sudden I couldn't walk more than five feet by myself, because the soles of my feet were cracked and bleeding, and the slightest pressure just killed me. I couldn't even tolerate the softest silk socks. And forget about wearing shoes. I lost my job selling dresses—not because of the time I missed, but because my boss said the appearance of my hands would revolt the customers. Thank God my husband left me enough money to survive on. The whole thing was like something I could have read in a book."

At the time Jonathan Harris began to come in, Arthur had begun to treat Bonnie using a UVB light regimen. Bonnie's feet began to clear enough that she was able to walk, but she still had a severe case of the disease. She came in for treatment every evening after work. If she missed a day, the skin on her palms and soles would grow thicker and thicker and then crack deeply.

When Jonathan Harris's biopsy results came in, it turned out that the lesion on the tip of his nose was a squamous cell cancer, those on his scalp were all actinic keratoses, and one of the ones on his ears was a basal cell cancer, while the other was benign. I explained to him the different ways we could treat the cancer: burning, freezing, radiation, surgical excision, or Mohs microscopic surgery.

"What do you suggest, Doc?" he asked.

Without hesitation I replied that Mohs microscopic surgery was the treatment of choice. I explained to him that Dr. Balin was so impressed by its results that he had spent a year living 5 days a week in Dallas so that he could become board certified in the method.

We made arrangements for Arthur to remove each of them, and then the conversation turned to what he considered his more pressing skin problem.

"Now, as far as my psoriasis," he said. "I've been dealing with this problem in one way or another for over half a century. Back when it first started, no one had any idea what caused it. They just knew the skin grew too fast. They must know more by now."

Several new theories attempt to explain how psoriasis develops. For years, it has been clear that the plaques of psoriasis result from an accelerated buildup of the skin's outermost layer and that there is an overgrowth of blood vessels below the plaques. In addition, the plaques themselves were known to be infiltrated with white blood cells. The difficulty has been in developing a hypothesis to explain all these signs.

One suggestion has been that psoriasis is due to a genetic abnormality, which would explain why it often runs in families. The new techniques of molecular genetics have made possible far more detailed explorations of the chromosomes and individual genes. Research groups around the world are approaching psoriasis from the genetic perspective. Already they have identified several candidate genes, which they are now studying in psoriatic individuals and families. While these studies may yield important new information about the role of inheritance in the development of psoriasis, it is likely to be some time before gene manipulation, either through replacement or inactivation of the "psoriasis gene," will become a viable, affordable way of preventing or treating psoriasis.

Another important theory that may yield a readily available therapy concerns the role of certain immune-system cells. A group at Rockefeller, headed by Dr. James Krueger, a contemporary of Loretta's, who was once a student in the Laboratory of Investigative Dermatology at Rockefeller, has discovered that psoriatic lesions have massive infiltrations of activated white blood cells, suggesting that an immune response has been mustered against *something.* The immune system is so complex and so intelligent that it almost seems to be a direct extension of the brain. Almost constant interplay and feedback occurs between the two, which may partly account for the apparent relationship between stress and disease susceptibility.

A number of immune-system cells attack foreign substances in different ways. Some of these cells, like macrophages, are nonspecific, meaning they will engulf and eat any foreign microorganisms that cross their path. There are T cells and B cells, both white blood cells. B cells are produced in the bone marrow and fight off invaders by producing antibodies. Immature T cells are synthesized in the bone marrow during early fetal life and then move to the thymus, a small organ underneath the breastbone, where they mature and learn their task of distinguishing between self and non-self. By adolescence, the thymus has shrunk and disappeared, but before doing so, it has programmed each of the T cells we each have at birth to recognize one specific antigen or foreign substance. When an antigen, like a virus, enters the body, inducer T cells, which are constantly patrolling the bloodstream, release a class of substances called *interleukins*. At least ten interleukins have been identified. All are involved in activating the immune system in some way. When T cells, which are normally in a resting phase, are activated, the particular T cell that has been programmed to kill a specific antigen that has entered the body is recruited. Within a few days, an enormous colony of these specialized killers is activated and available to do battle with the foreign substance.

Dr. Krueger's group found hordes of activated T cells in psoriatic plaques and almost none in healthy skin or psoriatic skin treated with PUVA. They discovered also that these activated T cells secrete interleukin-6, which has as one of its effects the ability to stimulate skin cell growth. In addition, the activated T cells themselves appeared to be attacking the psoriatic cells, which they were reading as foreign. When the researchers gave a drug targeted to bind to and inactivate these particular activated T cells, the psoriatic lesions healed, and the newly formed blood vessels disappeared.

Another promising idea that may help explain the typical psoriatic pattern of flare-ups and symptom-free intervals involves what are called superantigens. It has long been noted that latent psoriasis can be activated by various bacterial and viral infections; certain drugs, including antibiotics, antihistamines, and alcohol; and injury to the skin. Superantigens are toxins and other substances produced by invading organisms. But where most other antigens stimulate the proliferation of only those T cells that carry receptors specific for themselves, superantigens seem to cause a generalized stimulation of the immune system. Whereas antigens and their specific T cell receptors are frequently described as being like a lock and key, superantigens seem to function more like master keys, in that they can bind with T cell receptors for any type of antigen and turn them on. This can cause a huge increase of activated T cells in the circulation, all releasing growth factors capable of stimulating wild epidermal overgrowth or psoriasis. It is now thought that superantigens in the skin and bloodstream may serve to exacerbate or activate psoriasis in people with a genetic predisposition.

Yet again another theory, proposed by Dr. E. William Rosenberg, suggests that psoriasis is a defense mechanism against invading microorganisms. The location of the psoriasis lesions, he believes, may actually be indicating the presence of antigens that have entered the skin, either directly, from infected tissues, or through the bloodstream. Some proponents of this theory believe that psoriasis lesions often overlie the infected area and that, for instance, psoriasis on the lower abdomen may point to a pelvic infection or that psoriasis of the scalp may indicate sinus, throat, or tooth infection. There are those who say that the pustular psoriasis afflicting patients like Bonnie Williams is frequently triggered by yeast infections of the gastrointestinal tract. *Guttate,* or *eruptive,* psoriasis is often preceded by strep throat. Indeed, some cases of psoriasis do improve with long-term antibiotic or antifungal therapy to treat the underlying infection, either alone or in combination with PUVA or other standard treatments for psoriasis.

"That's all very interesting," Jonathan said after I had finished outlining these new theories to him. "Now tell me about new treatments."

"There are some new treatments, but many of the old ones work just about as well. Topical steroids are still the first treatment I would normally try, and I'm also interested in a new topical vitamin D derivative called calcipotriene."

Calcipotriene is sometimes referred to as "sunlight in a tube," because it, like sun exposure, increases vitamin-D-like molecules in the skin. Exactly how it works isn't precisely known yet, but one theory is that it slows down the overproliferation of epidermal cells and also may suppress activated T cells. Calcipotriene can be combined with ultraviolet light therapy, and the two together appear to have a synergistic effect against psoriasis.

"Although you had a bad experience with light therapy, we could still use it very carefully, to avoid burning you. You would have to come in several times a week for treatment."

"That would be hard," he said, "I work during the day, and most evenings I work as a literacy volunteer. Isn't there anything else?"

"There are also two drugs you take by mouth. One is called etretinate. It is related to drugs you may have heard of like Accutane and Retin-A. The other is called methotrexate."

Methotrexate, an anticancer drug, has been used to treat psoriasis since the late 1950s. It inhibits DNA synthesis in the rapidly dividing cells of the epidermis. Etretinate is a newer drug and has been used widely in Europe for treating psoriasis. Because they can be quite toxic, both drugs are reserved for patients with severe psoriasis that hasn't responded to other therapies.

"Dr. Pratt, the main thing is, I really want to try something that works this time. This is a bad outbreak, and it comes at a bad time, just as they always do. I really want to have more of a social life, hopefully even find an understanding lady friend. I can't come in for the light therapy because of my schedule, and the creams don't work well enough when I have psoriasis all over my body. I think I'd like to try one of those two drugs you just told me about."

I suggested he try methotrexate, since it is convenient and effective and it's been used more widely than etretinate in the treatment of psoriasis. Before he left that day, I drew some blood, so I could obtain a complete blood count and a biochemical profile. This would tell me about the health of his liver and kidneys. After he reached an effective dosage of methotrexate, I would send him to have a liver biopsy, so I could determine whether the drug was damaging his liver at all. Because of its effects on the liver, I told Jonathan he would have to refrain from drinking.

"That's not a problem," he said with a grin. "I went to AA back in 1966. I think I'd started drinking just a little more than was comfortable for my wife and me because it kind of helped me get through social situations. I finally got to the point where it wasn't helping anymore."

That night, Arthur and I arrived home at more or less the same time and were able to have dinner together. As it often did, our conversation turned to the day's patients.

"I referred a patient to you for Mohs surgery," I said. "He has a severe case of psoriasis as well as a squamous cell cancer on his nose and a basal cell on his ear and a couple of actinic keratoses on his scalp. I'm planning to treat him with methotrexate, and we need to coordinate, so I can hold off the methotrexate when you're operating on him."

"That lady I told you about with pustular psoriasis came in today after having missed almost five days of therapy because she had the flu. You wouldn't have believed how bad her feet looked. She had them completely bandaged, and even so, she was having such a hard time putting weight on them she had to be helped in by a friend."

Arthur had been treating Bonnie Williams for several months with UVB. He had spoken to me about her a couple of times. I knew she lived alone and had been devastated by the disease, with no one in the house to help her when her disease flared and she couldn't move around well. I thought about Jonathan Harris and his quest for a woman who could overlook his disease when it was so bad that the bed and the floor around his desk really did have to be vacuumed at least once every day. Clearly, their right to privacy prevented me from saying anything to either of them. But in my imagination, I couldn't help but introduce them to one another. Perhaps they would find enough common ground that they could be, if not life partners, at least good friends. It made me sad to think of their both coming to the office and never crossing paths.

"I wish there was some way they could meet," I said to Arthur. "I mean, here they both have the same problem. Maybe it would be a good thing for both of them. We ought to see if we can schedule them so they're in the waiting room together some time. . . ."

"Loretta," Arthur said, rolling his eyes in mock exasperation, "you're a doctor, not a marriage broker."

"I know. I didn't mean I'd go up and introduce them. I just thought maybe if they were in the waiting room together, they might strike up a conversation." I sighed. Arthur was right. It's sometimes heartbreaking to watch my patients' lives and know that, for the most part, my role is strictly to minister to their physical needs, when often I wish I could do more.

Jonathan's blood work showed up nothing that would prevent him from safely taking methotrexate. At his next appointment, I explained to him that he would start by taking a series of three methotrexate pills each week and that he should return to see me in nine days for another biochemical profile and blood count.

By the time he had received a month of treatment, the plaques on his elbows, trunk, and legs had improved considerably, but some fairly large areas remained on his stomach, hands, and arms. His blood count and liver and kidney function were still completely normal, so I increased his dosage slightly. Two months later, Jonathan's psoriasis was almost completely gone. The lesions that remained were small and widely scattered.

"This is incredible," he exclaimed. "I only wish I had met a doctor thirty years ago who was advanced enough to be using this stuff. Is there any chance of my being really cured?"

"You've responded very well," I said. "We might try reducing your dosage slightly sometime in the future, but, unfortunately, there's still no cure for psoriasis. Methotrexate is a good treatment, but you may need to keep taking it forever."

"If it keeps my skin looking like this forever, then I'm happy to take it. I feel ready to go out in the world again."

That was a year ago. Jonathan Harris comes in every few weeks for blood tests. So far, I'm happy to say, he has maintained his improvement.

Bonnie Williams's pustular psoriasis is presently under control with daily UVB treatment but, as she once told Arthur, "I feel that it's still there stalking me, and if I miss just one day's treatment, it starts to gain on me. It takes all my energy just to keep going."

I think the real tragedy of disfiguring skin diseases is that they so often deprive people of the human touch we all need to survive. I shudder to think of the cruelty inflicted throughout history and still continuing today in many parts of the world, as Chandrika's story makes clear. Jonathan Harris, although traumatized by the cruelty of his peers in school, was able to find an understanding woman once in his life. I can only hope that in his newly healed skin, it will be easier for him to find another companion.

Naked to the Light

⟐

It was the end of the day on a hot August afternoon. Loretta was already at home with our baby daughter, Allison. I had one more patient to see, but I was hopeful I would be able to dine with my wife and get to bed before midnight for the first time in many busy weeks.

One of the nurses put her head in the door. "Mrs. Sloan is waiting for you in room one, Dr. Balin."

Mrs. Sloan was a new patient. Glancing at the form she had filled out in the waiting room, I saw that she was fifty-five years old and the wife of a well-known orthopedic surgeon in the area.

My first impression of the patient who awaited me was that she looked at least ten or fifteen years younger than the age stated in her chart. In startling contrast to the many sun-damaged faces confronting me every day, here was the luminous milk-white complexion that hadn't been fashionable in over half a century. Clearly, this was a woman who understood how to care for her skin and had the self-assurance that allowed her to defy the still strongly felt preference for a summer tan. There would be no need to discuss with Mrs. Sloan the life-threatening danger of sunlight.

My dinner with Loretta seemed almost assured. I would carefully survey Mrs. Sloan, answer any questions she might have about caring for her skin, and be on my way.

"How do you do, Dr. Balin," she said, rising from her chair. "I'm glad to meet you."

As Mrs. Sloan extended her hand to shake mine, the sleeve of her dress slid back, and I was surprised to see a very large, very dark mole a few inches above her wrist. My heart sank. Although I couldn't be certain, of course, until I sent it out to be biopsied, it had all the outward features of a malignant melanoma, one of the most virulent and least treatable of all cancers. No matter how many times we see melanomas and other serious skin diseases, no professional armor lessens the sadness we feel upon meeting a patient bearing one of these potentially deadly emblems.

Dermatology is the most visual of all medical specialties. Where other physicians may need invasive instruments and esoteric imaging techniques to enter deep within their patients' bodies and listen to or see organs invisible to the eye, so much of what we treat lies on the surface, for all to see. Yet although they may be clearly visible to everyone, these surface signs are usually meaningless to all but trained eyes, as Mrs. Sloan so poignantly demonstrated. I could tell by her forthright and confident gaze that she was completely innocent of the cutaneous Sword of Damocles on her arm.

Struggling to control my expression so as not to alarm her, I said, "I see you're here to have your skin checked. Is there any particular concern you have?"

"Well, yes, Dr. Balin, there is. I feel sort of silly coming here, because I just saw my regular dermatologist back in May when I had poison ivy and she didn't mention anything amiss. But I was having lunch with a friend the other day, and she noticed this mole on my arm. I've had it for a long time, but I think it's a little bigger than I remember. My friend made me promise to have it looked at. I didn't go back to my own dermatologist, because I didn't want her to think I was questioning her. I know she saw it—how can you miss it?—but she said my skin was in great shape."

"Did your doctor do a skin survey when you saw her?"

"Well, if you mean did she look at all my skin—no. She just looked at the poison ivy on my legs, and she looked at my face."

"From what I can see, your skin looks very well cared for, but I want to ask you some questions, and then I'll do a complete skin survey. That's just routine in this office."

For the next twenty minutes, I asked Mrs. Sloan detailed questions not only about the mole that she had noticed—how long she had had it and whether it was changing—but also about her own and her family's medical history.

In the middle of the history-taking, she said, "I'm surprised at all these questions. I don't mind answering them, but what does heart disease and kidney disease and my parents' and children's health have to do with this mole?"

I explained to her that although this amount of detail might seem irrelevant to her skin problem, I would be uncomfortable doing an incomplete history and exam. Often, in the course of taking such a thorough history, I discover symptoms of diseases unrelated to the skin.

In our practice, every new patient, even those coming in for treatment of a simple rash, undergoes a meticulous examination of every inch of skin, including the scalp and even places rarely exposed to the sun, such as between the toes and under the arms. We do this wearing magnifying glasses that permit us to note very small spots that could easily be missed by the naked eye. We then take photographs for the patient's chart, so we can be aware of any changes that occur between visits. If we see something we don't like, it comes off then and there and is sent to a lab for biopsy. Our policy is not to let a patient with a potentially serious lesion leave our office until we have biopsied it. Sometimes a patient will come in with a mole or other presently benign growth that has the potential to transform itself and become cancerous. Such moles are photographed and then the patient is given a definite appointment, so we can recheck the mole in a couple of months. If there is any change whatsoever in the mole's size, shape, or color, then it will be removed at that time. Unfortunately, many people have gotten the idea from magazines and television that skin cancer is not in the same league as other cancers, like lung cancer and leukemia, and can be ignored. Indeed, skin cancers, when caught early, can usually be treated easily long before they have the chance to spread. But some *can* spread if left untreated, and they can even be fatal.

I left the room so Mrs. Sloan could change and went to call Loretta. It was clear our dinner together would have to wait.

I was fairly certain Mrs. Sloan did, in fact, have a melanoma. Her mole was large—nearly the size of a dime—irregular in shape, jagged at its edges, and an ominous mixture of red, blue, and black. Certainly I wanted to waste no time in removing it. If caught when still on the surface of the skin, a melanoma is as curable as any other skin cancer. But if it penetrates into the deeper layers, it can metastasize throughout the body. When this happens, it is virtually a death sentence. The cure rates are dismal. No presently known therapy can reliably stanch these dreadful tumors.

Even though we are taught that the unusual is routine in medicine, I was surprised to see a melanoma in someone whose skin appeared so pristine and undamaged. I put on my magnifiers and checked over every millimeter of Mrs. Sloan's skin. She had none of the typical stigmata of a sunbather—no wrinkles, no sagging jowls and wattles, not even any of the miscellaneous barnacles that often grow on sun-damaged skin. Nor did she at first glance appear to have many moles, another risk factor for melanoma.

"Have you ever had a sunburn, Mrs. Sloan?" I asked.

"Oh, heavens yes! I was an army brat, and my father was posted to lots of tropical countries. My mother always tried to keep us out of the sun—she was kind of old-fashioned in that way—but for a couple of years when I was a teenager, I sunned myself every chance I got. Unfortunately, with this white skin, I just cooked myself instead. I used to come home peeling and in so much pain I could barely lie down. But I never really got tan. Soon enough, I decided to give up and try to look like Marilyn Monroe instead. My husband says that's why I don't have very many wrinkles."

Loretta and I often say that if our therapeutic armamentarium contained only one weapon, the most lifesaving, as well as the most youth-preserving, would be the advice to avoid tanning. But whereas most patients are willing to listen to—are in fact clamoring for—advice on beautifying, improving, turning back the clock on their skin, so many resist this most urgent prescription in favor of quick fixes and after-the-fact repairs. To convince our patients to protect themselves in the sun is a far more difficult task than

convincing them to adopt other health measures, like quitting cigarettes or restricting their fat intake. No doubt this reluctance is a
product of mankind's ambiguous relationship to the sun.

Human beings have been sun worshipers since our earliest
forays from the caves. Every early culture had in its pantheon one
or more gods or goddesses whose symbol was the sun. As late as
the eighteenth century, Louis XIV, king of France, chose the sun
as his symbol and directed his subjects to regard him as the Sun
King—le Roi Soleil.

In Greek mythology, Apollo, the sun god, was also the god of
healing. Apollo's mortal son, Aesculapius, was said to be the first
physician. The staff of Aesculapius, entwined by a serpent, is still
the symbol of Western medicine. Indeed some of mankind's earliest scourges may have been partly conquered by the germicidal
power of sunlight, but like so many of our ancient beliefs that
evolved in response to real physiologic needs, worship of the sun
no longer serves us. Although sunlight has benefits—vitamin D
synthesis requires sunlight—long, unprotected sunbaths are not
necessary to provide this benefit. Only a few minutes of exposure
per day is adequate. Still, the association between sunlight and
health persists deep within the human psyche even today, when
the power of sunlight to wound and damage is increasingly
clear.

Many a modern-day Aesculapius, particularly those who, like
us, study the skin, has warned that the meeting of sunlight and
skin can be a dangerous, even fatal, encounter. Yet humans still
worship the sun, as a visit to any bathing beach will attest.

The fashion that encouraged tanning is comparatively recent in
the history of beauty. Until the 1920s, veal-white skin that appeared never to have seen the light of day was the standard of
beauty. Medieval ladies achieved the pallor fashionable in their
day by dusting their faces with flour and even by being bled to the
point of anemia. Later, women powdered their faces with a poi-
sonous white dust derived from lead paint or with crushed alabas-
ter. In an early version of a sunblock, they applied egg white to
their skin and even wore masks when they were exposed to sun,
lest a mole or freckle disrupt the milky beauty of their integument.
While her contribution to fashion may have been nothing short of
revolutionary, from our point of view, Coco Chanel must be re-

garded as one of the great villains of the twentieth century. It was she who made suntanned skin a symbol of chic rather than merely emblematic of a peasant lifestyle spent toiling under a hot sun. Soon it came to be that only those who worked indoors in factories and offices and didn't have the leisure or wherewithal to spend time in the sun were pale.

By the 1960s, Coppertone advertisements ("Tan, don't burn. Get a Coppertone tan!") and teenage beach movies celebrated a bikini-clad culture where a "deep, dark tan" was the essence of sex appeal. Cool teenagers were seduced by the cachet of a tan, and only nerds stayed lily white. Baby oil and aluminum reflectors were considered optimum tan enhancers, and sunbathers, basted in oils, lying atop aluminum reflectors, covered the beaches, backyards, and rooftops.

By the 1980s, however, the warnings of dermatologists and others in the medical community began to register. The first generation of sun worshipers was reaching middle age. The kinds of skin damage, even skin cancers, hitherto seen mostly in those who worked in the sun began to show up in people whose sun exposures had been purely recreational and cosmetic. Where fashion magazines once gave tips on perfecting a year-round tan, beauty editors began to extoll the "startling look of year-round pale skin." Advertisements for sunscreens began to crowd out those for Bain de Soleil and DeepTan, but consumers didn't budge. They continued to prefer what they considered a healthy, sexy glow.

"Your husband is right," I said. "You have beautiful skin. I would have guessed your age to be at least fifteen years younger, and you have the type of light skin that is actually very vulnerable to sun-induced wrinkling."

"Dr. Balin, this is what I don't understand. Even though my mother didn't agree, the teachers at school were always pushing us outdoors into the sun, and to me that makes sense. After all, primitive humans didn't have sunblocks. Why are doctors suddenly changing their minds?"

"Let me take a couple of photographs for your chart, and then you can get dressed and we'll talk in my office. Just knock on the door when you're ready."

Our patients often wonder why something as "natural" as sun can cause such harm. Surely we are meant to live in sunlight. After all, everyone knows we need sunlight to manufacture vitamin D. Most of us remember our parents urging us to go out and play in the sunshine. We grew up believing in its beneficence. Why, if it has the capacity to cause such disfigurement and even death, have human beings evolved in its light? When Mrs. Sloan was seated in my office, I said to her, "To understand why sunlight is harmful, you have to have a little education about sunlight."

Solar energy is transmitted the 186,000 miles between sun and earth as waves. The shorter the wavelength, the more energy it packs. Life on earth evolved in, and can survive in, only a small portion of the wide spectrum of energy emanating from the sun. The unamplified human senses can actually perceive only an even smaller portion of this spectrum: we can see some types of light, and we can feel the warmth of infrared energy. But the rest of the sun's powerful waves, like x-rays or ultraviolet waves, surround us without our being aware of them.

Ultraviolet light damages skin most seriously, although infrared, too, can cause problems: people who live in cold, damp parts of the world and must huddle next to stoves or fires develop a particular type of heat-induced skin disease. It is likely that some of the skin damage done by the sun can also be blamed on its heat.

UV light has several different wavelengths. The longest ones can penetrate the deepest into the body. When sunlight meets the skin, it is absorbed by molecules in the body called *chromophores*. An important chromophore in the skin is the pigment melanin, which determines skin color as well as how much we tan when exposed to sun. As sunlight hits the skin, it is absorbed by melanin and other chromophores such as beta carotene. As a result, less of the sun's energy is available to damage the genetic machinery of our cells.

"Where does the ozone layer come into all of this?" Mrs. Sloan asked. "Isn't sunlight somehow more dangerous now than it used to be because of the ozone layer?"

"The ozone layer is a thin band of gases above the earth's atmosphere. It's the first-line defense against those parts of the sun's energy that are harmful to life on earth. It's basically a protective mantle."

"So what's happening to it? What's this ozone hole I keep reading about?" She glanced at her watch. "I'm sorry. I'm asking too many questions and you're probably trying to get home. I know how my husband feels about chatty patients at the end of the day!"

Even though I was a bit tired and I really did want to see my family, I also wanted to take plenty of time with Mrs. Sloan. I was almost certain she had a melanoma, and this was a way we could build a working relationship before we had to get down to the serious business most likely confronting her.

"I'm happy to answer all your questions," I replied. "I wish all my patients were as inquisitive, because then I might really be able to make them understand about the sun. To answer your question about ozone depletion, the problem has to do with a class of chemicals called CFCs." These substances were first used as refrigerants and later as spray propellants for a variety of products from hair sprays to whipped cream.

Although CFCs were originally believed to be environmentally sound, because they are inert, nontoxic, noncarcinogenic, non-flammable, and noncorrosive, their inertness was what made them so harmful. Because they are not broken down, they are able to reach the ozone layer whole. When they do, they change the structure of the ozone.

"So you mean spray cans are going to destroy the atmosphere?"

"There is an expanding tear in the ozone layer." This tear is no small rip. When it appears, it covers an area the size of Canada. There are now predictions that as little as a 5 percent decrease in the ozone layer over the more densely populated parts of the planet will translate into a 10 percent increase in ultraviolet radiation and a dramatic jump in all types of skin cancers, including melanomas.

"So basically, you're saying that the hole in the ozone layer is letting more sunlight in, and that's why doctors have suddenly changed their minds about sun?"

"We're also learning so much more about what sunlight does, not only to skin but also to the rest of the body."

The major culprit in solar-induced skin damage is ultraviolet (UV) radiation, invisible and potentially deadly. Most people are familiar with UV in the context of "black lights" or the UV lamps used to kill bacteria in food-handling establishments. Many people now in middle age may remember being treated for acne under UV lights. Tanning beds also use UV light to produce an artificial tan. More recently, simple UV has given rise to a confusing alphabet soup of UVA, UVB, and UVC. (The latter are even higher in energy than UVB and are normally filtered out by our atmosphere. They're the type of UV light in germicidal lamps.) Sunscreens purport to block both UVA and UVB, while tanning-parlor operators frequently claim, erroneously, that they offer tanning under "safe" UVA lights.

Shorter-length UVB radiation has long been considered the chief culprit in sunburn. The SPF numbers on sunscreens that tell how long one can stay in the sun before burning occurs refer only to the effect of UVB radiation. Exposure to light in this region of the spectrum causes initial reddening due to dilation of the capillaries in the dermis. (The old-style sun lamps released only UVB light and, for that reason, never gave the appearance of a real tan. Twenty minutes' exposure to one of these left an all-over reddish cast but hardly the mahogany depth of a true Caribbean tan.) After the initial burning response, UVB causes delayed tanning, an effect that helps protect the skin from further photodamage. Delayed tanning occurs several days after the initial exposure as a result of increased activity or increased production of melanin stimulated by the UVB exposure. Darker skin provides greater sun protection, because it has more melanin to absorb UVB. Again, the amount of melanin determines the extent to which UVB tans rather than burns.

The majority of solar radiation that reaches the earth's surface is UVA. By itself, UVA does not burn the skin, except in long exposures—hence the shaky claims of the "electric beach" operators that UVA is safe. What UVA does do is produce an immediate darkening of the skin as it is absorbed by melanin. The purpose of this immediate darkening is sun protection. Thus, pale-skinned blue- or green-eyed Celts and others of British or Hibernian ancestry, who have low levels of melanin, don't experience an immediate pigment-darkening effect when first exposed to the sun, while those with medium or olive complexions and brown eyes do get immediate protective color as UVA reacts with the greater amount of melanin in their skin. Fair-skinned people are essentially naked to the sun. Not only does their skin contain little melanin, but they are constitutionally less able to step up their melanin production in response to UV rays. The intensity of color they can get is genetically predetermined, and no matter how long they broil themselves in the sun, their tanning ability is limited by their innate skin color.

If producing this immediate pigment darkening was all UVA did, tanning parlor proprietors might be somewhat accurate in their safety claims. Unfortunately, it is becoming increasingly clear that no UV exposure is safe. UVA can penetrate deep into the skin, disrupting the DNA and potentially leading to the types of genetic mutations that can cause the wrinkling and spotting and skin cancers we wrongly attribute to the toll of normal aging. As it blasts through to the deeper layers of the dermis, UVA injures blood vessels, causing the broken capillaries one often sees on the nose and cheeks of sun-damaged individuals. It can cause the destruction of elastic tissue, which gives the sagging, pouchy, wrinkled look we have also come to associate with aging but that is actually actinic (sun-induced) damage. UVA can also burn the eyes, resulting in cataracts over time.

Eventually a sunburn or suntan recedes, perhaps giving the impression that any damage that was done is gone forever. But skin, like film, is capable of enregistering light and storing it in its genetic memory, the DNA. With time as the developer, the memory of that light may emerge many years later, revealing its stored imprint in the form of wrinkles, liver spots, and other sun damage. When DNA is damaged by UV or some other agent, it may correct itself by means of one of several cellular mechanisms. The genetic damage may be repaired before it is carried on any further, like a run in a stocking that is stopped before it extends the whole length of the leg. However, if none of these repair pathways are activated, the future of the affected cells is unpredictable. A mutation in only one cell is all that is required to start a cancer. Precancerous lesions, like actinic keratoses, as well as all three types of skin cancers—basal cell, squamous cell, and melanoma—may all develop via this sun-triggered chain of events.

"I find all this so fascinating, Dr. Balin," Mrs. Sloan said. "I've never really understood anything about it before. I'm just sorry I've taken up so much of your time. Now, what do you think about my mole?"

This is the hard part. I enjoy teaching patients about their skin and how to care for it, but even though I see scores of skin cancers and even the rarer and more serious melanomas every week, I still find it painful to be the authority figure who has to break the bad news. I'd so much prefer to be able to say to all my patients, "Your skin looks fine. Come back in a year."

Instead, I heard my voice speaking the words I speak so many times a day: "Mrs. Sloan, it looks a little irregular. I want to biopsy it to be on the safe side."

"Biopsy it?" she gasped. "Doesn't that mean you think it's cancer? I just told you, I haven't been in the sun for thirty years."

I took her hand. "Let's get it off and then see what we have. We'll have a report in four or five days. In the meantime, I don't want you to worry."

Although I was fairly certain the lesion was indeed a melanoma, I wanted to make the waiting period as stress-free as possible for Mrs. Sloan.

We don't really know what causes melanoma, but there are a few clear risk factors. The most recent evidence implicates bursts of sun exposure and isolated blistering sunburns, particularly in childhood or adolescence. It is now widely held in the dermatological community that one severe sunburn before the age of eighteen doubles the risk of developing a melanoma. The incidence of melanoma is greatest in indoor workers and upper-income-bracket individuals, whose exposures tend to be brief but intense—the former because they try to maximize weekend and vacation tanning time and the latter because their vacations often take them to areas of maximum solar intensity, like the beach and the mountains. In contrast, farmers and others who work outdoors and spend many hours in the sun year-round are more likely to develop basal cell or squamous cell cancers as a result of their chronic exposure. While both types of cancer can be locally invasive and, if untreated, result in a fair degree of disfigurement, and although squamous cell carcinoma occasionally metastasizes these cancers are less dangerous than melanoma.

"So what's next for me, Dr. Balin?" Mrs. Sloan entreated. "What if it's a melanoma? Don't forget, I'm a doctor's wife. My husband has told me about melanomas. They're usually fatal, aren't they?" Mrs. Sloan looked deadpan, an expression I have come to know well in patients who have just been given this kind of news. Some people have a hard time processing the information at all, and others can't bear to let their fear show. I worry about patients like that. I often think of them leaving the office and driving home, alone with my words tumbling over and over in their minds. I try to spend as much time answering questions or just sitting with these patients as they need me to, although this, too, is sometimes difficult when I have a waiting room filled with patients nursing their own anxieties and wanting to get in and see me as quickly as possible. Rationing one's time in this way is one of the hardest parts of being a doctor. It's a bind not unlike that of working parents, who always feel they haven't given quite enough yet can't give more, simply because there are no more hours in the day.

"No, they're usually *not* fatal. If a melanoma is caught while it's still superficial, it has a better chance of a complete cure than breast or lung cancer or any of the other equally serious ones."

"But how soon can you find out for sure? I don't think I'll be able to sleep until you do."

"I want to remove your mole today, so that I can send it to Cornell for biopsy. I should have an answer in a few days, and we'll work from there."

Even though Alma Sloan's mole had all the hallmarks of a melanoma, there was always a good chance it was nothing more than a large mole with the potential to undergo malignant transformation. About 30 percent of malignant melanomas arise in existing moles. The rest are new growths. In this case, Mrs. Sloan had had the mole as long as she could remember. It was her impression that it had gotten bigger over time, but it had always been a dark, ugly—and, she felt, ominous—presence on her arm.

After the nurse had prepped the surrounding area by bathing it with antiseptic, I gave Mrs. Sloan an injection of the local anesthetic, lidocaine. As we waited for it to take effect, Mrs. Sloan spoke up: "Let's talk about melanomas. I can't really remember anything I've read about them, and it'll keep my mind off all these needles and scalpels."

The nurses had everything ready to go, so I sat on a stool facing

Mrs. Sloan. I started by reiterating that although late-stage, invasive melanoma is one of the deadliest of all the tumors afflicting humans, early-stage melanomas that haven't gone deep are one of the most curable. For this reason, a careful monthly self-survey of the skin must be considered in a league with breast self-examination as a preventive health measure. If everyone were informed of the dangers of unprotected sun exposure and knew the hallmarks of melanomas and other skin cancers, the death rate from melanoma and the disfigurement that occurs with other skin cancers would plummet, even as the number of new cases grows each year.

Instead, the melanoma statistics are alarming. A child born in 1994 will have a 1500 percent greater chance of developing a melanoma than a baby born in 1935. The death rate from malignant melanoma has risen 25 percent in the last decade, an increase greater than that of any cancer except cancer of the lung. How much of this increase is due to ozone depletion, how much to increased sun exposure, and how much to other factors is not clear. It is estimated that by 2000, one in eighty-seven Americans will, at some time, develop malignant melanoma. Of the approximately thirty thousand new cases of melanoma diagnosed each year, about six thousand will be fatal.

"Malignant melanoma is due to an overgrowth of pigment-producing cells," I told her. "Once a melanoma has formed, it can penetrate the layers of skin rapidly. If it goes that deep, it can come into contact with blood vessels and the lymphatic system and spread throughout the body." Melanomas can metastasize to any organ. Once they do, they carry a poor prognosis since no presently available therapies are reliably effective in inducing even a remission, much less a cure. But I was still hopeful Mrs. Sloan's melanoma hadn't invaded deep into her skin, so I decided against going into this worst-case scenario.

Melanomas appear earlier in life than other types of skin cancer, perhaps because their formation is related to intense, rather than chronic, sun exposure. While basal cell and squamous cell cancers normally appear in late middle age and beyond, 25 percent of new melanoma victims are age thirty-nine and younger. Melanomas strike both sexes equally, although they often appear on different parts of the body, depending upon sex. The most common sites are on the torso, back, arms, and legs. Women tend to have them on their legs more frequently than men, while men are six times as likely as women to develop a melanoma on the ear. Although not common, they do appear on the mucous membranes of the mouth and vagina, and even in the eyes. Melanoma is mostly a disease of light-skinned people. Whites have a ten times greater risk of developing it than do blacks. When blacks do develop melanomas, they often get them, for some reason, on the soles of their feet and under their nails—sites that are rare in other races.

Although the ultimate diagnosis of a melanoma depends upon removing it and examining it under a microscope, it is relatively easy to learn how to identify suspicious growths that should be looked at by a dermatologist.

Melanomas resemble normal moles but with some important differences. The *ABCD* system is a useful way to remember them. *A* stands for *asymmetry*. A normal mole is usually round, with both halves nearly identical. Most normal moles on the body are symmetrical, while a melanoma is asymmetrical. *B* stands for *border*. A normal mole usually has an even border with the surrounding skin. A melanoma often has a notched, irregular border. *C* stands for *color*. While normal moles are usually one color, melanomas are often many-hued. Although they are often black, bluish black, or dark brown, they may also contain areas of red, white, or tan. The edges may appear to bleed color into the surrounding skin. *D* stands for *diameter*. Melanomas are generally larger than the head of a pencil eraser, although we have certainly seen a number of melanomas smaller than this. Besides these cardinal signs, changes in size, particularly if sudden or continuous; changes in elevation and surface texture; and itching, pain, bleeding, and scaling are all signs that might indicate danger. Any such changes in an existing mole or the appearance of a new mole should trigger an immediate visit to a dermatologist.

When Alma Sloan said she could no longer feel the area I had blocked, I picked up a sterile scalpel and began the process of excising her mole for biopsy. Our standard procedure biopsying a suspected melanoma is to take a small rim of normal tissue all the way around the suspicious mole. This is done so that there is no possibility of cutting into the melanoma if this is what the growth turns out to be. If, however, the lesion turns out to be benign, we want to have taken off only what was necessary, since these excisions can leave large scars.

Sometimes, when a melanoma has invaded the skin, black pigmented areas are visible in the deeper layers, but this is not always the case even when the melanoma has already achieved a significant thickness. Sometimes the primary tumor may send out invisible threads of malignant cells that extend far beyond the visually apparent borders of the lesion. Melanomas may also spin off unattached satellite colonies of tumor cells in the area of the primary growth. So although I did not see any pigmentation extending down into the dermis, I knew that this was not *de facto* evidence of anything. When I had finished, the nurse put a dressing on the wound and instructed Mrs. Sloan in caring for it.

"I want you *not* to worry," I said to her. "If your husband is still in surgery this evening, is there a friend you could have dinner with? I think what you need at this point is dinner, maybe a glass of wine, and a good night's sleep. If you feel shaky and need to talk some more, here's my home phone number."

She smiled gratefully. "I really am pretty frightened. I know a lot of people with melanoma don't make it. I feel like I might as well just go into suspended animation until I know for sure. Charlie and I were planning a vacation. . . ."

"And don't you dare change your plans. This is just a suspicious mole." I promised her I would call her personally—she didn't want to hear the news from a stranger—as soon as I received the pathology report.

As I drove toward our home, the strip development ringing the city of Chester gave way to green pastures and fields of ripening corn. I was tired, and the peace of the countryside helped undo some of the tension of the day. Of all the skin problems I had seen that day—basal cell cancers, acne, rosacea, vitiligo, psoriasis, among others—only Mrs. Sloan's really frightened me. Anyone who has ever witnessed the velocity and the ravages of advanced melanoma can't fail to be chastened by the sheer violence of this tumor. I prayed that the biopsy report would come back negative.

Most melanomas are cured by straightforward excisional surgery or Mohs micrographic surgery. I nonetheless began to review in my mind some of the experimental approaches currently being tried in metastatic melanoma. Treatment of metastatic melanoma is difficult. Some of the newer approaches, which combine the current standard chemotherapy to kill the cancer cells remaining after excision with substances known as biologic response modifiers, to stimulate the patient's own immune system in fighting the cancer, seem to show some promise. These experimental protocols use either interferon, interleukin-2, or activated natural killer cells as immune modulators. The first two are hormones induced in various types of immune responses. Natural killer cells are a type of white blood cell responsible for disarming foreign proteins as well as, perhaps, burgeoning cancer cells.

The rationale for using immune-system boosters in addition to outright chemical exterminators or radiation is especially strong in the case of malignant melanoma, for there is evidence that melanoma may be one of the cancers amenable to destruction by an activated immune system that recognizes it and then deploys a barrage of antibodies and white blood cells of various types to overcome it. One of the features of melanoma that strongly supports such an interaction is the high rate of spontaneous regression of melanomas—the highest, in fact, of any cancer. The largest portion of all well-documented, spontaneously disappearing tumors has been in patients with melanoma. Presumably, this is the result of the immune system going to work and killing off the cancer without outside help.

Another approach being developed is a vaccine to immunize the patient to his or her own melanoma. This involves removing the tumor, preparing a partially purified extract from it, and then injecting it back into the skin. The rationale for this treatment is much the same as for any vaccine: the inactivated tumor antigens contained in the vaccine can trigger the immune system to fight off any remaining tumor cells. Another approach is to remove immune-system cells called lymphocytes from the melanoma and use them to carry drugs and other substances back to the tumor, which they are able to recognize as "self." While these approaches are theoretically promising, they are still only in the experimental stages and cannot yet be relied upon to save lives.

• • •

It was well after nine when I pulled into our driveway. Loretta had not yet had dinner, even though I had called from the office and warned her not to wait for me. Allison had only just been convinced to get into bed and stay put, and Loretta, who was pregnant with our second child, looked drained.

It was still light, so we took baskets and went out to the vegetable garden to forage for tomatoes and corn. The earthy, astringent scent of the tomato vines was bracing and reassuring. It reminded me, once again, of the physician's necessary connection to nature as well as to medicine. In the overwhelming desire to heal every patient who comes to us, both Loretta and I sometimes forget how important it is to spend this kind of time together when no one's life or looks or self-esteem is in our hands, when we're just a husband and wife in their garden. Like everyone, we need to recharge and gather our energies for our work. But because we are passionate about our work and because there is such urgency to much of what we do, it's difficult to take time off. Cancer cells are relentless in their pillaging of the human body. They don't take time off, nor do they need time to gather their energies. So as long as patients need our help, Loretta and I both have to fight the urge to work round the clock.

By the time we got back to the kitchen, we had already started to discuss Alma Sloan's case and some of the newer therapeutic regimens for melanoma that had been reported in the journals. Loretta reminded me of a heartbreaking patient I had seen several years before.

Dave O'Malley was a computer repair technician in his late twenties. He came to see me because of relentless itching that was literally keeping him awake at night. He arrived with a referral form from his HMO doctor stating that he had been treating Dave unsuccessfully for eczema for nearly a year. He had finally decided a one-time specialist consultation was perhaps in order.

Any dermatology resident could have seen from five paces that Dave didn't have eczema at all. His HMO had been spending money on rather involved treatment for eczema when, in fact, his problem was scabies mites, which could have been cheaply and easily treated. But Dave had more problems than scabies. In the course of examining him, I found a large blue mole on one shoulder blade.

"How long have you had this mole on your back?" I asked him.
"Which one?"

"This," I said, holding a mirror up to his back and pointing it out for him.

"Hmm," he said, a puzzled frown creasing his brow. "I think I've had *something* there for quite a while, but I don't remember anything that big."

I didn't like its looks at all. It had to be biopsied. I looked at the referral form from his HMO doctor. He had been sent to me for assessment of eczema only. I knew from virtually daily experience that it meant what it said. I had to get permission from his HMO doctor before I did the biopsy, or the procedure wouldn't be reimbursed. In fact, in doing the kind of careful once-over we do on every new patient, we are usually going beyond what we are authorized to do and what the patient's company is likely to pay for. Their argument is that general practitioners can take care of most problems for most patients, just as in the good old days, when the family doctor did most of the work and patients rarely saw specialists. I see this as a backward trend. Just as all areas of medicine are exploding with new knowledge, new diagnostics, and new treatments, insurance companies are doing their best to discourage subscribers from availing themselves of new lifesaving knowledge. There is no way any general practitioner can keep up with all this new information. He or she is occupied in keeping up on developments in family practice. It is completely unfair to ask these dedicated doctors to function as dermatologists, cardiologists, urologists, pulmonologists, and oncologists when they have neither the equipment nor the training and continuing education to do so optimally.

So in the person of Dave, we had a typical product of "health care reform": a young man with a highly suspicious mole that had been missed by a primary care doctor who, likely as not, didn't have more than a few weeks' rotation in a dermatology department during his internship year.

I explained the situation to Dave. He reached for his wallet. "There's a number you can call," he said, handing me a card.

It was a Saturday afternoon, and when I called the HMO, I was unable to reach anyone who was authorized to authorize me to do what was medically necessary.

I looked at the mole again. It just wasn't the kind of thing I could allow to leave the office, even if I had to swallow the cost of doing the biopsy and maybe even having it read by a competent lab. Loretta and I, and every other specialist in America, are finding ourselves in this annoying quandary more and more. And we have to remind ourselves more and more that as much as we care, we can't work for free. At one point, I seriously thought of shutting down our dermatology practice and just doing cosmetic procedures, which are unreimbursable and therefore don't involve insurance companies, to help us pay for the aging research. But even though we both resent being told how we can do our job by insurance company personnel and ultimately by politicians, there's no way Loretta and I could turn our backs on the scores of worried faces we see in our waiting room every day.

That day, I decided the mole warranted my biopsying it, no matter who paid for it. I asked Dave to wait while the receptionist continued to try to reach his insurance company. Eventually we got lucky, and I was able to get someone to fax me authorization to go ahead and perform the biopsy. In many cases, HMOs require patients to go all the way back to their primary care physician for his determination as to whether a specialist visit is needed. One might almost suspect a rather sinister corporate policy of discouraging visits to specialists by weaving people into a Kafkaesque labyrinth of bureaucracy. Unfortunately, on this occasion the company dictated that I send the biopsy to one of the labs they had under contract. This, too, is a distressing quandary we and many other dermatologists deal with on a daily basis. Not all labs are the same, and while most do a fine job of reading Pap smears or testing blood, few are set up to read skin biopsies adequately. For one thing, most labs employ a general pathologist to examine skin biopsies, but without specialized training in dermatopathology, these general pathologists are often unable to get accurate diagnostic information from the minute pieces of skin we send them. We have had so many serious problems with incorrect results that we now tell our patients we'd prefer to use a lab that is familiar to us and capable of assessing their particular skin condition accurately but that their insurance will most likely not pay for an out-of-network lab. If the patient wishes to use the insurer's chosen lab, he or she indemnifies us against responsibility for an incorrect reading by the lab. Most patients, like Dave that day, choose to pay to have their biopsies sent to a lab we know does good-quality work.

Dave's biopsy confirmed my worst fears. The tumor had invaded more than five millimeters deep (about a quarter of an inch). Even though I see several patients every year with melanomas this severe, Dave was one of the youngest. It was all I could do to keep tears from my own eyes when I walked into my office and saw him sitting there with the same expectant, innocent look with which so many of our patients greet us, knowing that in a few minutes his expression would change, and with it his whole world. One of the most upsetting tasks of learning to be a doctor is developing a way to tell patients, particularly young patients, that the tests have confirmed the worst scenario and watching the hope drain from their faces. It's not something that's really covered in our education. It's something we have to develop for ourselves, which explains why some doctors are so much better at it than others. You have to communicate a brutal truth without platitudes yet not rob the patient of hope, because hope is one of the most powerful tools in the doctor's arsenal. Patients who lose hope usually lose whatever chance they have for conquering a serious illness.

"Dave," I began, "I got your biopsy report back. The mole is a melanoma, and it's invaded a bit deeper than I'd hoped. I am going to remove a bigger area around it, and then I would like to get an opinion from an oncologist who specializes in the treatment of this type of melanoma. There are a couple of new options for treating invasive melanomas, and the doctor I'm going to refer you to is working with a new type of vaccine in addition to the standard treatments, which are chemo and radiation." I decided not to fill in between the lines just yet. What I didn't say was that although I would remove the entire primary melanoma itself, there was a high likelihood that the tumor had already metastasized. If it had, only radiation or chemotherapy could touch it—if, indeed, anything could at that point. The oncologist I would refer him to specialized in metastatic melanoma and had at his fingertips all the newest treatments.

When Dave left my office that afternoon, his last words were, "Pray for me, Dr. Balin." Those words echoed in my waking thoughts and in the moments before I fell asleep for days. They were powerful words. And I did pray for Dave, but my prayers weren't enough; the knowledge and skill of the oncologist weren't enough. The melanoma had metastasized. Over the next several years, Dave received the best treatments that modern oncology had to offer. Three years after his first visit to me, this brave young man was dead.

Like so many of the people we're seeing now, Dave had no notion of the sun's danger until it was far too late. He had spent his teenage summers lifeguarding and surfing at a nearby beach. He was out in the sun eight or more hours a day, and he never even wore sunglasses, he told me, much less skin protection. While I have always avoided the sun, even Loretta can remember going to the beach and baking, because it seemed like a healthy, relaxing thing to do after studying all week. By the time she had finished medical school, she knew more and was mildly cautious. On one of our first dates, we went sailing with my parents. Loretta, who had been ineffectually dabbing SPF 8 sunscreen on her face and arms, asked me to put some on her back. There was no way I was going to allow this woman I was falling in love with to be so inadequately protected. I quietly placed her sunscreen aside and brought out my own SPF 30. Loretta pretended not to notice the obvious change in texture as I applied it. "When you did that," she finally confessed, a year after we were married, "it was all I needed to know."

As the incidence of melanoma, especially in fair-skinned people, in areas such as Australia and other sunny parts of the world, began to rise, we stepped up our crusade against unprotected sun exposure. It was so clear to us that sun posed a major environmental threat—probably far more immediate than that of air pollution or contaminated water. We began to go out of our way to tell patients that the sun is a carcinogen in a class with cigarettes. And it doesn't just cause skin cancer.

Sunlight can also cause immune damage. Immunologists are now analyzing the results of more than two decades of studies on animals and humans, and their findings are chastening indeed. When foreign proteins like bacteria or viruses or irritants like poison ivy, known as antigens, come into contact with the skin for the first time, they are processed by specific immune-system cells in the skin, then presented to the immune system by a type of white blood cell known as helper T cells, and the immune system is activated. However, in some circumstances, an antigen may be presented to the immune system by *suppressor* T cells rather than *helper* T cells. If this happens, the immune system is specifically turned off to that antigen and cannot react against it. In other words, the immune system develops tolerance to the antigen rather than fighting it. In some cases, this is useful. One of the goals of immunologists working in the field of organ transplantation is to learn to manipulate the immune system selectively so it doesn't react against a donated organ, and immunosuppressive drugs are obviated. Clearly, however, if we were to develop tolerance to pathologic invaders like a virus, the virus could replicate unimpeded and cause great harm.

The newest bad news about sunlight is that it can destroy helper T cells and thus lead to a muted immune response. This can be a double-edged sword. If, for instance, a person encounters a new antigen—poison ivy, for example—for the first time following sun exposure, the poison ivy would be presented with suppressor, rather than helper, T cells, and the person would not respond to the poison ivy. In fact, the person would develop tolerance to poison ivy and never react to it.

Normally, our immune system is capable of detecting cancer cells and destroying them as they arise. However, suppose a cell undergoes malignant transformation just after a person has suffered a sunburn. If the new antigen (the cancer cell) was presented to the immune system immediately after the sunburn, when suppressor T cells were predominantly available, the individual could develop a tolerance to the newly formed cancer cell and would not be able to recognize and destroy it at an early stage.

Sun exposure may thus play two roles in the development of skin cancers. It may lead to changes in the genetic machinery that causes skin cancer in individual skin cells, and it may also kill helper T cells that would otherwise have recognized, fought off, and destroyed the skin cancer.

In short, there is simply no such thing as a safe tan. Tanning is a normal response to an attack by ultraviolet light, much as the formation of a callus is a short-term protective response to damaging friction. By its very existence, a tan indicates damage not only to the skin but perhaps to even more basic cellular structures. In an interesting new experiment, researchers took DNA that had been damaged in the laboratory and applied it to the skin. Amazingly, the damaged DNA alone was enough to cause the skin to tan without even a photon of ultraviolet light! This suggests that tanning is more than melanin's response to sunlight. It may also be an emblem of DNA damage.

Although we feel strongly about tanning, we also recognize that outdoor activities are important pleasures in our patients' lives. We don't tell them to avoid the sun altogether but simply to protect themselves when they go outdoors, and never to lie in the sun just to get tan.

Alma Sloan's results were faxed to the office a day later. The lab report read melanoma *in situ.* This meant that, unlike Dave O'Malley's melanoma, hers was still fully contained in the epidermis and was unlikely to spread, even though there is always the remote possibility that a single cell could have escaped into the circulation.

I was happy to be able to call her with the good news. "I want you to come in as soon as possible, so we can go back around the area and take off a little extra margin of skin to be sure no roots are left."

"I'm still scared," she said. "I wish I could feel completely carefree now, but I don't. Who's to say you really got it all or that there aren't other ones lurking in my body somewhere?"

"We did get it all, and as for any new melanomas that might appear, we're going to be keeping an eagle eye on you for the next several years. If another one develops, we'll take it off. I will want to see you every six months or so just to check that nothing new comes up and that any existing moles don't start to change," I said. "I don't want that to alarm you. We believe in being very conservative with something this serious, more conservative than many doctors might be."

"I'm just wondering whether Charlie and I should take that vacation after all. We were going to charter a boat in Florida for a week, but maybe I shouldn't."

"I have to tell you that I was very impressed the moment I saw you that you had managed to keep from getting any color at all, and yet you've told me you sail with your husband. It's clear to me you know exactly what to do to protect your skin—SPF 30 or higher, long sleeves, pants, and a big hat. You don't have to do anything more. Just keep it up."

"Yes, but I still got a melanoma. I feel like the only safe place for me is indoors. Maybe I can dare risk going out in the light of the full moon."

"Remember that melanoma is a freak of nature. Not all melanomas are sun related. It's entirely possible yours was due to a genetic predisposition rather than to your teenage sun exposures. Whatever factors actually came together to trigger your melanoma are probably long in the past. I'm not saying you couldn't develop another one, but I think you can feel confident your present level of sun exposure won't be to blame for it. And don't forget, we're all on the lookout now."

As Mrs. Sloan got up to see the receptionist for a follow-up appointment, I couldn't help but say to her, "By the way, I saw your husband sitting in the waiting room with you. He has a number of spots on his face that I can see. I really think he should be checked too. If he sails, he should be using as much sunscreen as you do."

She winked at this. "Misery loves company. I've certainly not had any success getting him to use a sunblock. Why don't *you* try? His idea of health is a good sunburn. And he's a doctor!"

Over the next several years, I saw Alma Sloan every few months. I removed one superficially invasive melanoma *in situ* from her leg and took off several suspicious moles, which turned out to be dysplastic, or precursor, lesions.

Because Alma spent so much time in our office, she became a dedicated proselytizer. If she saw a tanned teenager, she'd scold him or her and recount her own story. Once Alma had gotten hold of them in the waiting room, I found my patients much more receptive to my own tanning lecture. I would like to say Alma was equally successful with her husband, Charlie, but she wasn't. We removed several actinic keratoses, which are precancerous, from his face, ears, and hands, but nothing really convinced him to stick with his sunblock. At the beginning of each boating season he'd vow to be better, but then he would come for his checkup and say to me, "Look, Arthur, I wish I had known about all this way back when. But now the damage is done, and I'd rather be tan and wrinkled than gray and wrinkled. I promise I'll keep coming in to see you, I'll use the damned sunblock as much as I can, and I'll keep my fingers crossed." With other patients, I might try to convince them they could undo some of the sun damage by protecting it now and perhaps using Retin-A. In Charlie Sloan's case, all I could do was insist on regular skin surveys so that, with good luck, I could catch any new developments before they gave him trouble.

Alma Sloan's story is giving every indication of having a good ending, but we won't know for sure until she has been cancer-free for several years. Each time I examine her, I can feel her unspoken terror until I am able to give her the "all clear."

From our point of view, we can only hope the fashion that gave rise to tanning will be eclipsed by the sure knowledge that the sun is deadly and today's tan will be tomorrow's wrinkles and cancers. Over the years, cigarettes have gone from being a symbol of sophistication to one of ignorance. As one of Loretta's patients said to her, "Gee, Doc, first I had to learn to look sexy without a cigarette. Now I have to look like the pale nerds we used to make fun of on the beach." Perhaps the next decades will bring back into vogue the exquisite beauty of undamaged skin, so that only nerds will be tan. From our end, we can only continue to warn people of what lies ahead and hope we can convince them to stay safe.

A Vulnerable Shield

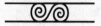

Ricky Mayfield was a backwoods boy whose desperate cry for help was heard a thousand miles away in the epicenter of medical sophistication, New York City. It came in the form of a letter written in a painstaking, childish hand on paper torn from a notebook.

"Dear Dr. Carter," it said. "My name is Ricky Mayfield, and I need your help, because I have EB. I have a real big sore on the top of my back, and I need to get it healed up so I can get me a job. My parents don't make much money, but they have been taking care of me since 1978. Please try and contact me as soon as possible, because it gets worse every day. Thank you, Ricky Mayfield." The letter was postmarked Argo, Kentucky.

EB, or *epidermolysis bullosa,* is the name for a group of diseases that render the skin so fragile that the slightest contact can cause it to become blistered and raw. EB is relatively rare, the incidence is between one in twenty thousand people and one in one hundred thousand to two hundred thousand, depending upon the type. All forms of EB but one are inherited, and most are present before birth. For babies afflicted with the more severe forms of EB, passage through the birth canal can be so abrasive that they are delivered into the world literally denuded. There is no way of handling such an infant that will not cause pain. Diapering, bathing, and even caressing are exercises in agony. And because, for these children, touch means only pain, they are deprived of the rich universe of learning only human touch can teach. In earlier times, the most seriously afflicted infants and children were shut away in back wards, because there was no help for them.

EB has three major types and twenty subtypes. The common denominator among them is that the layers of skin separate from one another, causing blistering and peeling. The mildest form of EB, *EB simplex,* occurs in the lowest level of the epidermis, the most superficial layer of the skin, and may not even manifest itself unless an unusual stress is placed on the skin and persistent blisters form. The more severe forms occur deeper in the skin. In the most severe form of EB, which occurs deep in the dermis, the raw wounds left after the blisters break do not heal well and are prone to infection and scarring. Chronic blood seepage from these areas can eventually cause anemia. The repeated blistering and scarring may result in skin cancer. While the disease is not fatal in and of itself, children with EB frequently die from severe infections.

These children are often very short and underdeveloped for their age. Malnutrition is a serious problem for them, since blisters in the mouth and esophagus may cause swallowing to be painful, and the teeth, which develop during gestation from the same embryonic layer as the skin, may be poorly formed or plagued with so many cavities that they require extraction. The lack of tactile stimulation forced by the extreme fragility of their skin can cause a deficiency of growth hormone release, which also contributes to stunted growth and development. To add to these young patients' misery are the frequent blisters in their intestinal tract and anus, which make even the discomfort of chronic constipation seem preferable to the agony of normal elimination. Occasionally, blisters in the intestines perforate, which can lead to sepsis, or systemic poisoning, and death. Malnutrition or the inability to move around comfortably often causes young patients to develop osteoporosis, the bone-thinning disease normally considered an affliction of postmenopausal women. In other words, children with severe forms of EB are small, fragile, and in nearly constant pain.

Putting Ricky Mayfield's letter in the pocket of my lab coat, I went upstairs to Dr. David Martin Carter's lab. He was sitting in a corner working on a grant proposal, while all around him research assistants and graduate students went about their business.

"What do you think about that kid's letter?" I began.

"I think we should invite him up here and try some skin grafts," he said. "It's his only hope to get that lesion on his back healed."

A t that time, Dr. Carter and I had been at Rockefeller for about five years. We had come down together from the dermatology department at Yale. Dr. Carter had been chosen to head a new joint dermatology service, the first department to be shared among the three great neighboring medical institutions clustered on Manhattan's East River: Rockefeller University, New York Hospital–Cornell Medical College, and the famous cancer center, Memorial Sloan-Kettering. This merger was undertaken to strengthen the dermatology department at New York Hospital, whose chief was planning to retire, and to ensure a future for Rockefeller's hospital. When Dr. Carter and I arrived in New York in 1981, we set about building the Laboratory of Investigative Dermatology at Rockefeller, writing grant proposals to fund the research we hoped to conduct there, and setting up a clinical dermatology service at New York Hospital–Cornell.

Prior to my arrival at Rockefeller, my longevity research at the Wistar Institute and the University of Pennsylvania had led me to develop methods for growing fibroblasts in the laboratory. Fibroblasts are the connective tissue cells responsible for the production of both collagen and elastin. I had chosen the skin as the organ in which to study aging, because it is the most accessible and easily visualized organ system and one that clearly shows various types of damage and time-related changes.

Whether from the skin or any other organ, all normal cells have a finite life span. (This is not true of cells that have undergone malignant transformation. They are immortal.) When removed from the body and put into flasks, cells are capable of dividing only a limited number of times. After this they do not die, but they are no longer able to proliferate, and I wanted to know why.

Clearly, some sort of built-in program determines how long cells live. Cells obtained from a newborn or a fetus live longer than cells obtained from an adult. To understand some of the mechanisms and the biochemistry of this change in proliferative capacity might yield important clues to the aging process, ones that might call into question the inevitability of aging, even of death. Our bodies are masterful self-healers. Each of our cells has repair mechanisms and self-maintenance programs running twenty-four hours a day. Not only are these self-protective and self-healing mechanisms efficient, but we're making and exchanging atoms within individual molecules all the time. So many individual parts are constantly regenerating, yet the whole runs down. If indeed a built-in program limits cellular life span, we have to understand it to see if we can modify it, and I wanted to discover what conditions and events might prolong cellular life span to its maximum potential. To do so, I learned how to grow cells, so I could expose them to specific environmental conditions and observe how they behaved.

Looking back, I realize that although I had planned no clinical application for my cell culture techniques, my later decision to apply what I had learned about growing cells probably originated back in my medical school days. Medical school is, for most future doctors, their initiation into the realities of doctoring. Although I, like many other pre-med students, had spent time working in labs and hospitals, it's in the third and fourth years of med school that one is first presented with seriously ill patients and really comes to know firsthand the unique jubilation of triumphing over illness or injury and also the incomparable sense of defeat when one can't save a person.

I still carry around in my memory pictures of a little boy named Jimmy Jaacks, who was helicoptered into the trauma center at Penn with second- and third-degree burns over most of his body from a fire that had engulfed his parents' trailer. Healing from massive burns like his is slow and painful. When such large areas of skin are destroyed, healing, which proceeds inward from the outer edges of the burn, often causes the skin to contract and cause disfiguring or even disabling scars unless a graft is placed over the center of the wound.

In those days, the most commonly used grafting technique required the painful removal of patches of skin from unburned areas of the patient's body, which were then placed on the burned areas. Not only was this an excruciating process that usually involved multiple operations, but in some cases, the result was visually appalling. In Jimmy's case, so little healthy skin was left to work with, his doctors decided to use sheets of skin removed from cadavers to shield the burned areas during the healing process. The most difficult problem with this technique and others that use foreign tissue, like pigskin or human amniotic lining, is graft rejection. But even in cases where the graft survives the immune system's attempt to destroy it, the foreign tissue never merges with the patient's own skin and it never grows. These grafting techniques offer at best a temporary covering.

Although Jimmy was being treated in a special burn unit and wasn't under my care, the whole hospital was aware of his plight. We all heard about the many disheartening setbacks as his healthy young immune system fought off graft after graft. Over the years, until I started at Rockefeller, I saw other gravely burned patients, many of them children, but somehow this early exposure remained most vividly in my mind. At the time, I knew what was needed was a better type of autograft, one harvested from the patient's own body but that didn't require the painful removal of large areas of the patient's remaining healthy skin. A living bandage cultured from a small number of the patient's cells was what was really needed.

After medical school, I began to experiment with ways to grow skin cells in culture. At that point I was focused on improving my culturing technique, so as to provide myself with plenty of skin cells for my experiments. I wasn't thinking about using the sheets of cells for grafts. Yet as so often happens, the basic research spun off unpredictable clinical applications.

When I arrived at Rockefeller, I found that a researcher by the name of Jack Hefton, across the street at Sloan-Kettering, was developing similar culture methods to produce skin for use as burn dressings. Together we developed a technique to culture skin cells, starting with only a very small piece of the patient's own skin. In some cases, we used the small, flesh-colored growths most people have on their necks or underarm area known as skin tags. In others, we used a suction device to create a small blister on the patient's skin. After removing the roof of the blister and separating out the cells we wanted to grow, we put them in a flask containing a special nutritive stew of culture medium and skin growth factors we had developed. After a few weeks, we would have sheets of epidermis ready for grafting.

Cells grown by our method attached better than other types of grafts. The self-grafts seemed to speed the healing of the underlying tissue. Moreover, they released skin growth factors of their own that also stimulated the patient's skin to grow.

By the time these studies began, I had been studying the growth of human cells in culture for ten years. One of my experiments studied how oxygen influences cellular growth and cellular life span. I was fascinated to find that oxygen is actually toxic to cell growth. In fact, cells make a host of biochemical responses in an attempt to defend themselves against oxygen. Room air, which contains 20 percent oxygen, is not optimal for fibroblast or melanocyte cell growth. Most types of skin cells, whether in culture or healing wounds, grow best at oxygen levels similar to those in most of the body—about 1–2 percent oxygen, although epidermal cells flourish at 10–20 percent oxygen. At Rockefeller, we found that fibroblasts grown at lower oxygen concentrations not only grew faster, but also lived longer in culture. Studying how human cells responded to an oxidative stress allowed me to explore the importance of free radicals and reactive oxygen species to the aging process.

We continued to search for ways of enhancing cell growth, so as to develop new models in which to study the biology of aging. But because we were in a clinical setting at the Rockefeller Hospital, we also used the cell culture system to try out new approaches to common dermatologic problems like wound healing. Our findings flew in the face of the traditional medical dogma that healing wounds benefit from plenty of fresh air. Instead, we found that wounds heal much faster if kept moist and under an airtight dressing.

At the time we received Ricky Mayfield's letter, we had just received funding to begin a new clinical study using the laboratory-grown skin grafts to treat children with EB and to start an international registry of EB patients.

After our conversation that morning, Dr. Carter contacted Ricky and learned his story. Ricky was born in 1964, and although it was evident at birth that he was afflicted with EB, at that time little could be done to help children with this disease, beyond making them as comfortable as possible. Ricky was never brought home from the hospital. Instead, he lived on a ward for the first fourteen years of his life, seeing his parents only during an occasional visit. "It was okay," he told Dr. Carter. "The nurses and doctors were my family." When Ricky was fifteen, he was sufficiently stabilized to go to live with his family on their farm, miles from the nearest town. In anticipation of Ricky's arrival, his family rearranged the house, installing for the first time an indoor toilet.

Although his condition had improved enough to permit his moving in with his family, life for Ricky was painful and lonely. His clothes stuck to his raw skin, and he suffered from frequent infections. His mother, who worked in a nearby mill, was ashamed of her son's appearance and never took him to town. There were no close neighbors in the isolated hollow and, except for his loving grandmother, Ricky had no friends.

By this time, Ricky had developed a deformity typical of severe EB, in which the hands become so encased in scars produced by repeated blistering that the eroded skin between the fingers eventually fuses. In such cases, the bones are often reabsorbed, leaving a useless mitten, a process and a result not unlike the bound feet of a Chinese lady. Ricky was unable to participate in most normal activities, and he was unmercifully ridiculed at school. But after all he had suffered, such cruelty couldn't break his spirit. "They all tried to push me around," he said, "but they underestimated me."

Ricky attended his high school graduation on a stretcher, with a raging fever from his infected wounds. Soon afterward, the doctor who had been treating him since birth read about our laboratory at Rockefeller and the EB registry and mentioned it to Ricky. But it was Ricky who took it upon himself to write to us and ask for help.

Ricky Mayfield had the most serious form of EB, which occurs in the deepest layer of skin. Although it is not the most common, it is the most widely studied form of the disease. In this type of EB, it is thought that the blisters may form because of excessive collagen breakdown. In normal skin, an enzyme called collagenase, which breaks down collagen, plays important roles in skin growth and wound healing. However, patients with the most serious forms of EB may produce four times as much collagenase as normal. Not only is there more of it, but it appears to be abnormal in structure. In Ricky's type of EB, dystrophic EB, the anchoring fibrils, formed from a specific type of collagen, which normally connect the basement membrane beneath the epidermis to the dermis, are lacking. Without these anchors, the skin is vulnerable to blistering and shearing. The layers of the skin can separate like damaged veneer.

Recently, scientists have been able to identify the mutations and individual genes involved in certain forms of EB. Because of these advances in understanding these genetic aspects of the disease, babies with EB can be diagnosed as early as eleven weeks after conception via chorionic villus sampling and the obstetrical team prepared for a particularly gentle Caesarean birth. But none of this information was available when Ricky was born.

Walking on Rockefeller's riverside campus, in the middle of Manhattan, one feels at the very heart of the mystery and grandeur of science. Big Science—the kind that wins Nobel Prizes. In fact, Rockefeller is sometimes referred to as the "Nobel Farm" for the large numbers of laureates nurtured there. The Rockefeller Institute for Medical Research, founded in 1901 by John D. Rockefeller Sr., was, at one time, the most important clinical research center in the United States. Its hospital, generously equipped, and staffed by the best minds money could attract, was responsible for the majority of medical research undertaken in this country before 1940. It was at the Rockefeller Institute's hospital that the three blood groups were first identified, where DNA was discovered to be the genetic material, where the first heart-lung machine was built. But by the 1960s, less and less research was being conducted there, and the hospital was in danger of closing. It was no longer the institute's visual and intellectual centerpiece. Rockefeller had grown to encompass wider areas of scientific investigation. By the mid-1970s, Rockefeller had become the most important mecca for basic science in the nation. No longer just a research institute, it was now a full-fledged university.

How far away from Argo Ricky must have felt as he walked past Rockefeller's gatehouse on his right, the sky-blue dome of the auditorium on his left, and up the hill toward the ivy-festooned Founder's Hall. Although he had arrived in New York City with a paper bag containing enough clothes to last him the three or four days he assumed he'd be staying, Ricky was to live in room 323 at the Rockefeller University hospital for nearly nine months.

On Ricky's first morning at the Rockefeller hospital, Dr. Carter and I came in to visit him just after he had finished his breakfast. We were both curious to meet this courageous boy who had come so far to seek our help.

Although Ricky was actually twenty-two at the time, like most young people with severe forms of EB, he looked many years younger than his chronologic age. He still had the stature and unbearded face of a prepubescent boy. Despite his crippling disease and the obvious pain of his many wounds, he greeted us with a cheerful smile.

"I wish I could shake your hands," he said ruefully, "but I can't." He held up his two scarred mitts. The left hand, which was the more tightly bound, had no fingernails and more closely resembled a club than a human hand. Although the four fingers of Ricky's right hand were curled tight, his thumb was still free, and it was by virtue of this remaining digit that Ricky had been able to write to us. I thought with amazement of the long journey he had taken by himself.

"Good morning, Ricky, I'm Dr. Carter, and this is Dr. Balin. I know you've come a long way to see us, and we're going to do everything we can to make you feel better," Dr. Carter said, taking Ricky's scarred hand in both of his. "I want you to understand that you're an important part of the team. We're going to do this together. Okay, partner?"

"Yes sir," Ricky replied, his blue eyes immediately engaging. He was an appealing kid with a thatch of blond hair and a mischievous glint in his eye.

The first thing we did was examine Ricky's entire body. Blisters and weeping sores covered much of his skin. Both his arms and legs had a number of smaller blisters and wounds in various stages of infection. His entire back from buttocks to shoulders was raw. He looked like an animal that had been skinned and left to dry in the open air.

"It doesn't look like these sores have been dressed for a while," Dr. Carter said, as we surveyed the vast expanses of exposed flesh.

"No, I can't reach my back too good," Ricky said apologetically. "When I lived in the hospital the nurses used to put bandages on me, but my mother didn't want to touch me." During the day, he said, his clothes would stick to his open wounds, and, when taking them off in the evening, he would invariably tear off large strips of skin. Even if the disease weren't continually producing new blisters and open wounds, his skin could never have healed in the face of such unremitting daily trauma.

"Ricky," Dr. Carter said, "we have a way of covering some of these sores that ought to help them heal, but sometimes it can take quite a while—maybe even six months or more. Can you stay away from home that long? You can live here in the hospital, and it won't cost you anything."

"Oh sure, I can stay. They don't really want me at home with all these sores on me anyway. Maybe if you can get them healed up, they won't be so disgusted with me."

Dr. Carter nodded at me. "Dr. Balin is going to explain the treatment to you."

Ricky turned expectantly to me. "What we have been doing for people with EB and certain other diseases, Ricky, is to take a tiny piece of their skin and grow it in the laboratory so that it gets big enough to use as a kind of bandage. Because it's your own skin, we think it's the best way to heal your sores and make new skin grow. After you've had a couple of days to settle in here and we've done some tests on you, we'll start. What we'll do today is put Vaseline dressings on your sores. That ought to make you a lot more comfortable, and you won't have any more problems with your skin sticking to your clothes."

"That sounds good to me, Dr. Balin, sir."

And thus began Ricky's transformation.

For the first few days, Ricky soaked in cool oatmeal baths to soothe his raw, itching skin and help remove some of the crusts that had formed over his blisters. After his bath, a nurse would spend several hours carefully dressing his skin with the Vaseline-covered bandages. Then Ricky was free to roam the floor for the rest of the day.

It would be impossible to overstate the contribution made by the nursing staff in caring for Ricky and the other children with EB. These were healers in the highest sense of the word. We worked as a team dedicated to using all our shared skills and knowledge to mend these wounded children. While we covered their wounds with grafts grown by dedicated technicians and other members of the research team, the nurses healed with the loving touch of their hands and the beneficence of their presence.

At that time, one or two other children with EB also lived at Rockefeller, and several others came in for treatments. In his first week at Rockefeller, Ricky met and befriended Scott Bachko, our first EB patient. Scott was five years old and, like Ricky, had been diagnosed at birth. When Scott first came to our floor, his face was so covered with erosions that he looked like the victim of a severe burn. The wounds never had a chance to heal because, night after night, Scott would scratch them so violently in his sleep that by morning, his face was once again raw and bleeding. The repeated blistering and healing had caused facial scars that pulled his eyelids down, making it impossible for him to close his eyes normally. As a result, he suffered constantly from dry, irritated eyes. After making the rounds of several pediatricians who were unable to help, Scott was referred to a dermatologist in his hometown, Salt Lake City. Unable to heal Scott's wounds using a variety of special dressings and pigskin grafts, his dermatologist contacted us.

When Ricky arrived, Scott was living in the hospital with his mother, who slept on a cot next to him so that she could try to keep him from picking at his face. Ricky soon became like an older brother to Scott. Ricky, who had never known family life, seemed delighted to have this adoring young sidekick. Scott, for his part, revered the older boy. Often the two could be seen together, watching television or listening to records in the dayroom. Ricky also took it upon himself to spend time with Scott's mother, telling her about his own lifelong experience of what her son was undergoing. As time went on, Ricky became quite good at talking to other patients and their parents. For the first time he was listened to and taken seriously, his disease no longer a barrier between himself and others but, rather, a bridge.

After Ricky had been in the hospital a few days, we decided he was ready for us to begin his skin grafts. At that time we had a new clinical scholar in the lab. Her name was Dr. Loretta Pratt, and she had just finished her internal medicine residency. One of her jobs was to obtain fragments of skin with which to begin the grafting process. Using a suction device left in place for about twenty minutes, Loretta raised a small blister on healthy skin in the center of Ricky's chest and then carefully removed the top of the blister with a scalpel.

After Dr. Pratt had removed the roof of the blister, she took it to the lab, where it was processed to separate the epidermal cells. These were then put into flasks containing a standard cell growth medium, to which we had added certain skin growth factors newly available in those days. From these few cultured cells, Ricky's living bandage would begin to grow.

It took about three weeks to grow a sheet of skin about four or five inches in diameter and several layers deep. When it was time to transfer the new skin to Ricky's back, I pressed a Vaseline-coated piece of gauze over the sheet of skin and placed it skin-side down onto his exposed dermis. Then I covered the graft with a sterile pressure dressing to hold it firmly in place. Our earlier studies of skin healing had convinced us of the importance of dressing wounds with an occlusive bandage that kept the wound moist. Within four or five days, the implanted skin would begin to merge with the raw skin beneath it.

Ricky's back had such a large area to be covered that we maintained a continuous cycle of raising blisters and growing and grafting skin. Fortunately, some of the contents of each tissue culture flask could be used to seed new flasks, much as fresh batches of yogurt can be produced from residue from a previous batch, so we didn't have to raise a new blister each time we wished to produce more material for grafting. Although we probably had the best technique in the country and the best contamination control, from time to time we would lose a growing culture, as a result of contamination somewhere along the line from bedside to finished product. This would become apparent because the culture medium would begin to cloud over with pillaging bacteria, which would eventually use up the growing medium for their own nourishment, killing the burgeoning skin cells. We would then have to throw that batch away and begin again. Fortunately this was rare.

At the same time we were grafting the wounds on Ricky's back, we were also grafting areas of Scott's face. In Scott's case, only his face was severely afflicted, but where it had struck, the disease had created a horror mask that was at once gruesome and pathetic, with erosions distributed like a clown's red grease paint on the tip of his nose and his cheeks. Although Ricky had a more severe form of EB and much more extensive involvement, the disease had been less cruel to him. In sparing his face, it had permitted him to present himself to the world with a smile that most often was mirrored back to him in the faces of strangers. For Scott, the eyes of strangers too often registered shock or repulsion, or else they looked right through him, as if he didn't even exist.

Another young EB patient referred to us at about the same time was Diego Jackson. Diego, like Ricky, had been born into a poor family, but unlike Ricky's mother, who was repelled by her son, Diego's young mother looked at her horribly disfigured child with the beatific expression of an Italian madonna cradling her holy infant. Every day was a fight against dispiriting odds. Diego's father, an alcoholic and off-and-on heroin user, hadn't been seen since soon after Diego's birth. His mother struggled to support him and his older sister without resorting to welfare. To manage, she juggled a night shift at a fast-food restaurant and a job as a mailroom clerk in the mornings. The family lived with Diego's grandmother in one of the projects at the north end of Central Park. We saw little of this young mother, not because she was a bad parent but, indeed, because she was such a good one.

"I know my baby's in good hands here," she told Dr. Carter soon after Diego had settled in. "You're looking after him better than I can for now, but he's always in my thoughts and prayers. Right now I'm just concentrating on getting ahead, so I can give Diego and his sister some kind of future."

Diego's disease was not diagnosed until he was a year old. The first sign was merely a small blister on his neck. Within a month he had developed more blisters on his back, groin, and legs. Diego's mother took him to one doctor after another, but none was able to diagnose this rare disease nor make the blisters heal. By the time Diego was finally referred to a dermatologist at Columbia-Presbyterian, his face was a mass of ulcerating blisters whose seepage merged with his continual tears of pain, resulting in nearly unbearable itching and irritation.

When Diego came to live at Rockefeller, the disfiguring disease had ravaged his body for eight years. Like Scott, he could not fully close his eyes, and his orbits were red and raw. Countless cycles of blistering and scarring around his nose had caused his nasal cartilage to collapse and his nostrils to become occluded, forcing him always to breathe through his mouth. From a distance, he looked battered and flayed.

Although he had been an eager learner at the Head Start program he was entered in, he lasted only a few months in first grade. The other children—and even some of the parents and teachers— were so horrified by the little boy's appearance that they shunned him like a leper. As they became used to him, the children's screams of terror turned to jeers and taunts, which were more than Diego could bear on top of the unrelenting pain of his disease. Within a few months, the outgoing little boy he had been vanished, and Diego became so withdrawn and inaccessible that it was decided he would wait a year before trying school again.

Away from the mocking judgments of their unblemished peers, these three boys began to heal emotionally as well as physically, but it was a slow process. For the first several months of his stay, Diego remained in his room with the door shut, clutching a much-handled teddy bear. Loretta and the floor nurses would have to coax him to open his door and join the others in the playroom. Ricky, on the other hand, was outgoing and enthusiastic about life, against all odds. He used the eraser tip of a pencil to hit the keys of a typewriter to write. With a pencil he held in his teeth to draw, he began to make cartoons for his fellow patients and some of the staff. Dr. Carter, whose own children were grown, had a number of Ricky Mayfield originals on the walls of his office.

After a series of grafts, the skin on Ricky's back began to heal, and we were starting to make progress on his arms. Rather than trying to place the grafts contiguously, we placed them in different areas of his back, with the hope that they would form outgrowths of their own and begin to merge with one another. The grafted areas healed over well. Although they didn't look like pristine new skin, in that they were paler and more translucent, they reduced his pain and prevented his clothes from sticking to his back.

"Ricky, I should think you might be wanting to get back home," Dr. Carter said to him one morning during rounds.

"Yep," was Ricky's only reply, and then he looked away. (Later, he was to tell us that he had begun to think of Rockefeller as home and, since he hadn't heard from either of his parents during the many months he had been up north, he had begun to wonder whether he would be welcomed on his return or whether his parents might have decided he was "more trouble than I was worth.")

"We'll want to see you again in a few months, but I don't see why you shouldn't go home for Christmas."

And so, in mid-December, one of the nurses accompanied Ricky to Port Authority and put him on a bus bound for Knoxville, Tennessee, the closest city to where he lived.

Scott and his mother were themselves anxious to get home in time for Christmas. After several attempts at grafting the wounds on his face and having him dislodge them in the night, we had devised something resembling a football helmet to shield his healing skin while he was sleeping. Most children might have balked at wearing this rather uncomfortable nightcap, but Scott's mother had the good idea to tell him to pretend he was an astronaut who had to keep his space helmet on at all times. By the time Ricky left to go home, Scott's erosions were healing nicely as the newly grafted epidermis began to meld with identical cells in Scott's skin.

Then one morning as I was sitting in my office, preparing a slide lecture on oxidative stress and skin cell growth to present at an upcoming conference on the biology of aging, I got a call from the head nurse on Scott's floor.

"Dr. Balin, we need you down here right away. Scott fell on his face, and we've got a mess."

I arrived on the floor to find Scott sitting quietly in his bed, blood seeping out from beneath his grafts. His mother was weeping.

"Oh, Dr. Balin, I don't know how it happened. Honestly, he was playing in the dayroom, and I was watching him and reading, and the next thing I knew he had fallen right on his face, and of course he hasn't been having to wear his helmet during the day. Now what's going to happen?"

I took the small face in my hands. So far, there hadn't been much damage. The grafts had healed completely, and the fall hadn't dislodged them. But we couldn't be sure what their fate would be until we saw how much swelling might occur and whether the trauma would set off a new round of blistering.

"Fortunately, the grafts had a chance to heal well before this happened," I said. "We'll dress them and, with luck, they'll stay intact."

"But he wanted to be home in time for Christmas so badly," his mother wailed.

"And chances are he won't be disappointed," I said. "Let's wait and see."

By the next morning, blisters had appeared on the grafted areas. I feared this was going to be a severe setback. In the worst case, all the blisters would ulcerate and destroy the graft. But to everyone's delight, the situation got no worse. By the time Scott left for Salt Lake City two weeks later, the blisters had healed completely, and the grafts were holding. We had made arrangements to consult with his local dermatologist as needed. Since, so far, only his face had developed severe blisters, we were hopeful the rest of his body might be spared. We were not to see Scott again for five more years, and when we did, it was in quite a different setting.

Ricky Mayfield returned for another round of grafts in February. By this time, large areas of his back were beginning to fill in with healthy skin. Although the areas that had been severely eroded would always bear scars, gone was the raw, weeping surface. Of course, the treatment did not prevent the formation of new blisters. Ricky would need treatment and daily nursing care for the rest of his life.

The next step in helping Ricky was to send him to an orthopedic surgeon at New York Hospital, where he could have surgery to release his hands. Since the individual fingers are usually still present within the scar tissue, surgical degloving may be able to separate them. Unfortunately, new blister formation may cause the fingers to re-fuse within a few years, necessitating repeated degloving operations. Ricky's surgery was only partly successful. The thumb and forefinger and ring and little fingers of his right hand were freed, but to this day, those of his left hand remain fused and useless. Because of the risk of re-fusion of the fingers of his functioning hand, Ricky must always pay special attention to the areas between his fingers, having them bandaged or even splinted apart whenever new blisters form on his hands.

Diego's face was healing well following eight grafts. Although Diego was African-American, when he arrived it would have been impossible to discern his race on the basis of his facial skin, because there was none, and we are all the same color below the epidermis. By midwinter, after he had been in the hospital nearly a year, some of the pigment had returned with the healing of his skin. His face was so well healed that we decided it was time to send him to New York Hospital for surgical correction of his eyelids and reconstruction of his nose. Both operations were successful. As his skin healed, so did his spirit. In fact, a mischievous streak began to emerge, much to everyone's delight, despite the fact that he was often quite naughty. Diego discovered, for instance, that there was fun to be had by filling latex examination gloves with water, tying them closed, and dropping these five-fingered bombs onto cars passing below his window on FDR Drive. As he began to feel more at home, he began to hoard food in his room and decorate every surface with pictures of Michael Jackson and other stars. Dr. Carter, with his intuitive kindness and empathy for every human and animal in his surroundings, knew Diego needed a father figure. He would often deliver mock-stern lectures to the boy about the sloppiness of his room. "We *don't* hang our clothes up on the floor," he would say. Or "This room looks like a dress rehearsal for the Battle of the Bulge, Diego!" But although his criticisms were delivered with good humor, Diego understood Dr. Carter meant it when he told him to clean up his room with particular respect to the banana peels he often draped on his bedside table and the bubble gum wrappers that littered every surface.

After Ricky had been back with us for a couple of months, we noticed a persistent reddish plaque on his forearm that was clearly not a blister. Because patients with EB are prone to develop skin cancers, I biopsied the lesion and found my suspicions were correct. Ricky indeed had a squamous cell cancer. Unlike those that often arise on sun-damaged skin in the fourth decade of life and beyond, the squamous cell cancers that occur in EB can be aggressive and metastasize widely and rapidly, often ending in death. Originally it was believed these cancers resulted from the generalized trauma to the skin that occurs in EB lesions. More recent research has suggested that mutations in one of the genes involved with collagen production may cause patients like Ricky with recessive dystrophic EB to lack tumor suppressor genes, inborn cancer preventers, normally located nearby on the same chromosome. If these findings are borne out, it may someday be possible to predict which EB patients are likely to develop these aggressive cancers.

Although we were able to scotch that first cancer, we were still worried that more might appear. As with all these young patients whose disease may cut short their lives, we hoped to do as much as we could with our skin grafts to give Ricky a chance at a normal life and some happy years.

Because Ricky was the oldest of the EB patients, he had the most freedom to come and go, and gradually he began to enlarge his boundaries. First he began to walk around the Rockefeller campus, which extends six blocks along York Avenue. Unlike many urban campuses, Rockefeller has lawns and tall trees and views of the East River, and it is protected from the outside world by a wrought-iron fence and a gatehouse. As he gained confidence, Ricky began to venture out into the safe neighborhood beyond Rockefeller's gates, which consists largely of hospitals, doctors' offices, and former tenements that now house medical students and hospital personnel.

Ricky returned once more to Kentucky in the early summer, with an appointment to return to Rockefeller after Labor Day. When he came back in September, we noticed that he brought more baggage than he had on previous visits. He carried a large knapsack on his back, and hooked in the fold of each elbow was a shopping bag.

"You're coming along, Ricky. The grafts have been holding well, so you probably won't have to stay here more than a month this time," I said, feeling pleased that our work had been successful and that Ricky could go home to his family at last.

But to my consternation, tears began to course down Ricky's cheeks. "It ain't my home," he muttered. "But I guess you're telling me this ain't my home either."

"But Ricky, don't you want to go back and be with your cousins and your grandmother? I know you and your mother aren't getting along well at the moment, although that may change. But you told me you love your grandmother."

"My grandmother's dead. She died while I was away, and my family don't want me around. Those people ain't my family. They don't know how to treat me right. They make fun of me. Please, Dr. Balin, can't I stay here? Please?" He clutched at my hand with his two stumps and hung on tight as sobs wracked his thin frame.

When I told Dr. Carter about the scene in Ricky's room, he said, "If he wants to stay up here, let's see what we can do to help him."

Within two months, the social workers at New York Hospital had found Ricky a small room in the shadow of the 59th Street Bridge and arranged for him to begin receiving SSI payments, which would cover his living expenses. He came to Rockefeller every day to have his wounds dressed, and he continued to enjoy spending time with Diego and some of the new patients. When another graft was required, he would move back into his old room at the hospital until he was sufficiently healed to undergo outpatient therapy.

Soon after Ricky moved out, I decided to seek additional training in Mohs micrographic surgery. To do this, I had to leave Rockefeller and spend a year at Baylor Medical Center in Dallas, Texas. It was time to start to realize my lifelong goal of building my own research institute, where I could devote more of my time to aging research. Seeing patients and doing research, the two complementary parts of my professional life, are always in a shifting balance. Although most of my time during the Rockefeller years was spent doing research, I had also been seeing dermatology patients in my father's office in Chester, Pennsylvania, near Philadelphia, every weekend. I had started using one room in his office while I was a resident in dermatology and pathology at Yale. Subsequently I took over the whole building on Providence Avenue, where he had practiced for over forty years. My ultimate plan was to open a practice in Mohs micrographic surgery and cosmetic dermatological surgery in Chester. I hoped that by doing so, I could establish my own research laboratory and assume the majority funding of my aging research without depending on government grants.

Curiously, there is little funding for longevity research in our youth- and beauty-obsessed country. I was beginning to find that I was spending more time writing grant proposals than actually doing the research or seeing patients. When grant money did come through, it was usually for one year at a time. So just as I had trained technicians and postdoctoral fellows in my techniques and had the study up and running, we would be running out of time and money. Often the grant would be renewed, but not until a year or two later, during which time I had had to let my trained personnel go. When the new grant money came, I would be faced with starting from zero. In the end, I realized, I would be better off setting up my own lab and paying for my own research, even though that would mean working double time.

I had persuaded Dr. Pratt to join the practice. I was glad she had agreed to come, because I found I was growing very fond of her. Besides, she was extremely capable, both in the lab and with patients. My own feelings for her aside, I knew she would be a perfect addition to the practice.

In 1991, Dr. Loretta Pratt and I were married. When I think of the series of coincidences that brought us together, I realize it was Dr. Carter I had to thank. A chance meeting between his brother, the Reverend Dr. James Carter, and Loretta in a Chinese restaurant across the street from Mount Sinai Medical Center brought her to Rockefeller. Loretta had run around the corner to grab some food on a break from her hectic medical school schedule. Seeing this pretty girl with a stethoscope slung around her neck, Dr. Carter's brother had asked her whether she was a nurse. No, a doctor, she had replied. Dr. Carter's brother, a Presbyterian minister from St. Paul, Minnesota, was having lunch with his young niece. He had actually chosen to strike up a conversation with Loretta because he was trying to demonstrate to his niece that not every stranger, even in New York City, was dangerous and to be avoided—that some were, in fact, kindly and interesting. When the conversation revealed that Loretta was planning to be a dermatologist, he told her that his brother, Martin Carter, was setting up a dermatology research lab at Rockefeller and that she ought to go up and meet him. This was in 1982. Loretta remembers that I showed her around the day she came to visit, but I have no recollection of it. And that might have been considered our beginning. I don't really know where it began for her. Even as a Clinical Scholar in our lab, Loretta always seemed a somewhat ethereal presence. I would no sooner catch sight of her at the end of a corridor or filing out of a lecture than she would vanish. This, she later explained to me, was wholly intentional, because she felt that every chance encounter with me ended with my mentioning some new idea I'd had that would require her to stay up even later at night, growing yet another batch of cells in the lab. For that reason, she rarely joined the rest of our group at lunch if I was there and seemed to find a way of ducking into fire stairs and ladies' rooms every time she caught a glimpse of me. Eventually, she came to think of me as something other than a slave driver, and we became fast friends as well as highly compatible colleagues.

Early one morning in 1994, the telephone rang. Loretta answered. From where I stood drinking my morning coffee, I could see two tears waver at her eyelashes and roll down her cheeks. When she hung up, she turned to me with a look of sorrow I will never forget. "Dr. Carter is dead."

On the train to New York, we saw several other dermatologists headed to the funeral. Because of numerous delays all the way along the line, we reached the church just after the funeral service had begun. Inside, it was standing room only, but we managed to find two seats in the balcony. When we were seated, Loretta, who had been very quiet for the entire trip north, suddenly began to sob quietly. Following her gaze downward, I saw why. The first three pews were filled with Dr. Carter's young EB patients. They were all there: Ricky Mayfield, who by that time had lost the lower part of his arm to more cancers, and Diego Jackson and his mother. Even little Scott Bachko, now ten years old, had come all the way from Salt Lake City. And there were others—children I hadn't treated. Some were in wheelchairs, many were heavily bandaged, some were amputees—children so thin and small and in so much pain, one marveled at the great love that had brought them to say good-bye to this man who had given them hope, a man described in his *New York Times* obituary as "a prince among men."

Sitting next to my wife, gazing down from that balcony onto the heads of the brave children below, I silently blessed the man who had brought us together as the chords of "All Creatures of Our God and King" swelled in the air around us.

POSTSCRIPT

We still keep in touch with some of our patients from those days. Ricky Mayfield still lives in the same room near the 59th Street Bridge. He is over thirty now. After Dr. Carter died, his Laboratory of Investigative Dermatology was continued by Dr. Jim Krueger, whose interests lie in understanding the causes of psoriasis. Ricky's blisters are now treated, when necessary, with cadaver skin grafts rather than sheets of his own skin, but for the most part, he thinks they work quite well. Every other day an aide comes to dress any active sores. The rest of the time he is free to enjoy the corners of the city he has made his own. His best friend is a bouncer at the Hard Rock Cafe, Ricky's favorite New York night spot. He has several friends who take him for drives in the country, and he still sees Diego, who now has an apartment of his own in Brooklyn and is finishing his long-deferred high school education by correspondence. Diego's mother is an executive secretary at a large insurance firm.

Ricky continues to have problems associated with his EB. He developed a tumor on his knee, which was removed. Shortly thereafter, another tumor developed in his throat. Recently, we received the sad news that Scott Bachko, age fifteen, had died from a rapidly metastasizing skin cancer.

These are the harshest realities of this dreadful disease, but hope is on the horizon.

An important development has been the introduction of prenatal diagnosis, which can be done via either amniocentesis or chorionic villus sampling. Several types of EB can be diagnosed in this manner.

The ability to identify specific gene mutations through DNA studies allows a much more precise identification of disease subtypes. For instance, the tests can now tell a woman of childbearing age whether she is carrying the gene for dominant dystrophic EB, which her chances of passing on are fifty-fifty, or for recessive dystrophic EB, for which the risk is many times less.

The identification of the specific mutations involved in several forms of EB provides a foundation that someday, with luck, will lead to gene replacement therapy, in which defective or missing genes can be reinserted into the patient's DNA. Gene therapy is the ultimate treatment goal for most serious genetic diseases.

While we do not have any patients with EB in our practice at the moment, every time I read about one of these new developments, I think of Ricky and hope that, in his lifetime, a specific gene therapy will become available and that he will be near the head of the line of those waiting to receive it.

The Mind's Hieroglyphs

"Every practitioner, therefore, who studies the honour of his profession and the happiness of his patients should assiduously endeavor to cultivate an acquaintance with the anatomy of the mind as well as that of the body."

W. WOODVILLE, 1788

One morning as I passed through my waiting room, on the main floor of the building Arthur and I share in Chester, I noticed a striking Asian woman whom I assumed was my first patient of the day. Her makeup was deftly applied, and she was wearing a well-cut black linen suit and black-and-white spectator pumps. The only item of clothing that seemed inappropriate was the black wool turban she was wearing on that hot, late-summer day. I wondered whether she was perhaps undergoing chemotherapy and had lost her hair, but her eyebrows and eyelashes, which also would have been affected, were full and natural. I nodded good morning to her and passed through the waiting room into my suite of examining rooms.

"Is that my first patient in the waiting room?" I asked my secretary, Pam.

"Actually, she isn't. You have Mr. McNally, then Jenny Ackroyd, then Mrs. Dyson, and *then* her. Her appointment isn't until eleven."

"Is she aware of that?"

"Oh, yes. She said she wanted to be sure she was on time."

I thought this a little odd, but I assumed she had come from a long distance, as many of our patients do. "Why don't you offer her a cup of coffee or tell her how to get to the deli, since she's going to have such a long wait."

"I already offered her coffee, but she says she never drinks it."

"I wish I could fit her in earlier," I said, glancing at the morning's schedule, "but she's a new patient, and I'll need to spend some time with her." Since I had a few minutes before my nine o'clock patient arrived, I scanned the medical history form each patient fills out. The woman's name was Nancy Cheng. She was fifty and married, with three children. She had once been a nightclub singer, but she had recently retired and now worked as a freelance voice coach. Her only complaint was hair loss. I was surprised to see that she had not checked any of the boxes pertaining to cancer history. Nor was she taking any medication that might cause alopecia, or hair loss. She was taking a long list of nutritional supplements, including some Chinese herbs, and using Rogaine lotion on her scalp.

When Nancy's turn came, I entered my office and found her sitting on the edge of her chair, leafing through a hairstyling magazine. On her lap, next to her purse, lay a small white paper shopping bag.

"Good morning, Mrs. Cheng. I'm Dr. Pratt," I said, shaking her hand. "What brings you here today?"

"I'm losing all my hair," she said, pointing to the turban. "It's getting to the point where I can barely face people. And at the rate it's falling out, I won't have any hair left at all in a few years."

I went over her history with her. She denied having any of the health problems, like thyroid or pituitary abnormalities or lupus, that can cause hair loss. Although her seventy-year-old mother had slightly thinning hair, Nancy said her own hair loss was already far worse. She had visited several other doctors, but they had all been "useless." The last physician had prescribed the Rogaine.

Rogaine, known generically as minoxidil, was actually developed as an oral antihypertensive medication. When patients taking it for high blood pressure began to report that it made hair grow on their foreheads, it was reformulated as a topical lotion to treat scalp hair loss. Although Rogaine has serious side effects when taken internally, it is generally safe when applied as a lotion. It is

hardly a miracle cure for baldness. It produces cosmetically significant hair regrowth in only about 15–20 percent of patients, and
even if it makes the hair grow, the new hair may be only vellus
hair, the soft, fuzzy, nonpigmented hair of an infant. Moreover,
minoxidil seems to be useful only for early baldness. It will not
transform a longstanding bald pate into a bushy head of hair. But
even in cases where it doesn't actually grow new hair, minoxidil
almost always stops or slows down further hair loss. Although
how minoxidil works is not really known, one theory is that it
increases the blood supply to the scalp and thus raises the skin
temperature. In time, these changes may make hair grow faster
and possibly increase the diameter of individual hairs.

"Because this is your first time here, Mrs. Cheng, I want to
check all your skin very carefully. My nurse will bring you a gown.
Please remove all your clothes, except your underpants, and of
course I'll need you to remove your turban."

"Okay," she said. "But you're going to be shocked."

And shocked I was when I entered my examining room a few
minutes later, for even standing next to her and looking down at
her scalp as she sat on the table, I could see she had a full head of
glossy black hair.

I wasn't quite sure how to respond to what I saw. As far as I
could tell, Nancy's purported alopecia was a figment of her imagination. Such patients are not uncommon in dermatologic practice.
They are something of a problem, because in treating them, one
must tread a fine line between corroborating with their perception
or telling them nothing is wrong and losing their confidence. Accordingly, until I am certain that there is no physical basis for such
a patient's complaint, I say nothing about my doubts and proceed
with the same thorough diagnostic workup I would use if the
patient's problem were as obvious to me as to him or her.

"When did you first notice that you were losing your hair?" I
asked.

"I'd say it started about three years ago."

I probed her scalp carefully. Although at close range her hair
could be seen to be slightly thin, it was hardly abnormally so. I
took a comb and ran it gently through her hair, letting it part in its
natural place. The width of the part, a useful indicator of excessive
hair loss, was only marginally greater than normal. "You *appear* to

have a pretty normal head of hair, but of course this is the first time I've met you," I said tentatively.

"If you had known me ten years ago, you wouldn't say that," she said with a wry laugh. "I'm just trying to hold on to what's left. Every time I wash my hair, I lose a huge amount, and I have to be very careful not to pull any more out when I brush. I never have permanents or do anything that might hurt it. I even wash it with very diluted baby shampoo." She reached down and brought the shopping bag up to the table. "Look in here. That might give you an idea of how bad this is."

I opened the bag. Inside were two large fistfuls of black hair.

"That looks like a lot," I said, "but it's a little hard for me to assess. What I need you to do is a more controlled hair loss census. Before you leave today, I'll explain to you how we usually do that."

She nodded, clearly pleased that I was now taking her complaint seriously.

"How long have you been using the Rogaine?"

"Well, the last doctor I saw prescribed it for me in March, but I didn't really want to use it. Then about two months ago, it was obvious I had to do something. I started losing so much hair, I was terrified that I really was going to go bald. So I filled the prescription, and I've been using it since then."

"Did you notice an improvement after you started using it?" In fact, it takes many months before Rogaine's effects are apparent, but I wanted to find out as much as I could about her own sense of reality.

"Not really. I don't think it's even working. That's why I'm here. You came highly recommended, and I hoped you'd have some tricks up your sleeve."

"First we have to find out what's making your hair fall out. There are a number of reasons for abnormal hair loss, and of course the treatment will depend upon the underlying problem."

Hair is made of elongated filaments of keratin, the same waxy protein found in the epidermis, nails, and tooth enamel. It grows from follicles, which are actually extensions of the epidermis. We are born with all the hair follicles we will ever have. Some follicles are genetically destined to grow long, pigmented hairs, known as terminal hairs, while others grow short, fine vellus hairs. Examples of terminal hair are scalp and eyebrow hairs, while the more ethereal vellus hairs cover most of the body and are often invisible to the unaided eye.

Scalp hair grows in a cycle consisting of a two- to six-year growth period followed by a transitional resting phase that lasts for a couple of months. At any one time, approximately fifteen percent of the one hundred thousand or so hairs on the head are resting, while the rest are growing and lengthening. During this resting phase, a hair stops growing, separates from its root, and develops the small, waxy, club-shaped tip that many people mistakenly assume to be the hair root. After this "club hair" is shed, a new hair shaft begins to form in the same follicle, and a new cycle begins. During the club, or *telogen*, phase, hairs are not attached to the scalp by a root, and they can more easily be pulled out in the course of brushing, washing, or styling. It is perfectly normal to shed up to one hundred resting-phase hairs a day.

That is the normal cycle. However, abnormal hair loss has other causes. Probably the most common is overproduction of male hormones called *androgens*. In males, androgens are responsible for the typical male body hair pattern and male sexual development. In females, androgens produced in the ovary and adrenal gland determine hair growth and body hair patterns. Androgens must be present for excessive hair loss to occur in either sex. Eunuchs, for instance, who have virtually no male hormones, retain luxuriant scalp hair into old age but have little body hair. What is fascinating and still mysterious is the fact that the same androgenic stimulation that causes men to lose their scalp hair over time also seems to stimulate the growth of other hairs. Typical of the aging male is the sprouting of ever coarser hairs from the nose and ears and the softening and lengthening of hair in the pubic and underarm areas.

After I had checked the rest of Nancy Cheng's skin, which was in good shape, with little sun damage and no worrisome moles, I asked her to get dressed. Back in my office, I explained how I wanted her to collect and make a careful count of the hairs she shed each day. Since most people who believe they are losing hair perform this ritual anyway, they are usually delighted to comply when their doctor asks them to continue doing what they have been doing all along in guilty secrecy.

"I'd like you to take a fresh envelope each day for a week, date it, collect all the hairs that fall out, count them, and put them in the envelope. Take a week off, then collect and count them for one more week. That will give me a chance to observe your hair through most of a month, and I'll be able to see more clearly how your hair responds to your hormonal cycles and whether the shedding gets worse or better. I'd like to see you back in three weeks. In the meantime, I want you to discontinue the Rogaine until I get a better idea of what is going on. Before you leave, I'll ask my nurse to give you some literature on hair loss that I think you will find interesting."

"Oh, thank you, Dr. Pratt," she cried. "Thank you so much for taking me seriously! I don't really think those other doctors believed me. Even my husband says he can't see any difference in my hair. He thinks I'm being silly, but men . . . what do they notice?"

When Nancy returned, we tallied up each day's hair collection. The numbers ranged between eighty and one hundred—nothing extraordinary. When many hairs are in the resting or telogen phase, it is quite normal to lose one hundred or so hairs each day.

"So what do you think, Dr. Pratt?"

"This doesn't appear to be grossly abnormal," I said. "A certain amount of daily hair loss is entirely normal, Nancy. Lots of people lose this much hair every day, but most aren't as observant as you are. You should be aware, too, that in this type of climate, people shed more hair from about September to December, so you may be moving into the time of year when your hair loss would normally increase."

She looked deflated and unhappy that, once again, her complaint was being downplayed.

I went on. "The next step is to draw some blood and to do a scalp biopsy. The blood work will tell me whether you have a hormonal imbalance that could account for your problem, and the biopsy will allow me to find out more about the health of your follicles."

When women begin to lose abnormal amounts of hair, it is usually due to hormonal imbalances, childbirth, or the use of certain medications that affect the endocrine system. Trauma inflicted on the hair in the name of beauty is another frequent culprit. (One way to distinguish between hairs lost to normal shedding and those lost due to styling or processing damage is that, in the latter case, hairs do not have a club at the tip, because they are being broken off along their shaft.)

If female alopecia is due to excessive androgen production in the ovaries, it can usually be reversed by giving the patient either birth control pills containing estrogen or else prednisone, a steroid. Hair loss in women can also be caused by deficient production of androgen-binding globulin, a protein produced in the liver. This globulin attaches to androgens circulating in the blood and inactivates them. Underproduction of androgen-binding globulin may result from estrogen and thyroid deficiencies. If this is the underlying problem, it can be treated with thyroid medication, birth control pills, or the type of estrogen replacement given to women at menopause. Hair loss can also be caused by excessive skin sensitivity to male hormones. Occasionally, the hair follicles contain too many receptors for androgen. This, too, can be treated with birth control pills, to lower the amount of androgens in the blood, or with spironolactone, a medication normally used to treat high blood pressure, which can block androgen receptors so that they can't receive and respond to the male hormone.

"But a biopsy is going to make it even worse!" she protested. "Then I'll have a bald spot forever."

"No, Nancy, I promise you that won't happen. First of all, I remove a tiny piece of your scalp, and I'll take it from one of the thinner areas. After I've closed it with a couple of stitches, which will be invisible in a few weeks, you'll see that the thin spot has vanished."

"I wish you didn't have to do it," she said. "But I trust you wouldn't do it if it weren't going to tell you something." With a resigned sigh, she removed the beret she was wearing.

In my examining room, I anesthetized a small area on the crown of her head, removed a minute piece of scalp, then sutured the incision.

"I'd like to keep those envelopes of hair," I said, "so I can have a closer look at them."

"All right," she said, clearly edgy at parting with her hair. "But please guard them with your life."

"I certainly will," I solemnly agreed.

A closer examination was needed to rule out the possibility of a condition called *telogen effluvium.* While doctors had observed for hundreds of years that some patients could lose large amounts of scalp hair seemingly overnight following such bodily traumas as high fevers, shock, hemorrhage, and certain drugs, and sometimes even in the aftermath of severe emotional stress, no one knew why it occurred—just that it did. It wasn't until 1961 that this sudden hair-loss syndrome was named and elucidated by Dr. Albert Kligman, the world-famous dermatologist at the University of Pennsylvania.

Dr. Kligman discovered that such sudden hair loss is caused by an abnormal increase in the percentage of hairs in the resting phase at one time. Instead of the usual fifteen percent, fifty percent or more of the hairs are resting and thus are candidates for shedding. After two to four months, these hairs begin to rain down in large numbers—as many as a thousand each day—for six or eight months. In many cases, even this level of shedding is virtually invisible to others. I thought there was a reasonable chance this diagnosis would account for Nancy's symptoms.

Later that evening, I examined the hairs I had plucked. Only twenty percent or so were in the telogen phase, eliminating the possibility of telogen effluvium as a neat explanation for Nancy's symptoms.

Two weeks later, when the blood test results were back, Nancy returned to the office.

"What the blood work shows, Nancy, is that you do have a very mild hormonal imbalance. What's happening is that your hair's growing cycle is getting shortened, and the resting phases in between growth cycles are becoming longer. The name for what you have is androgenetic alopecia." I could see she was reassured that I could identify what she had.

"There are several treatment options, but before I discuss them, I do want to say that I'm concerned you may be worrying too much. Anxiety can really make the problem worse. Your test results are basically reassuring. You have mildly thinning hair, but it's highly unlikely it will ever get much worse. Certainly you shouldn't fear going bald."

"But when you say *anxiety,* you're not trying to tell me this is all in my mind, I hope."

"Absolutely not. I'm saying that anxiety and stress really can contribute to hair loss. The stress response is hormonal, and it can exacerbate the slight hormonal imbalance that is causing your hair to thin."

Patients like Nancy present a quandary. I was still skeptical of any physiologic basis for her complaint. No one, looking at her, would ever think to say her hair was anything but an enviably sleek fall of beautiful Asian hair, without so much as a thread of gray. Her blood tests were borderline. To say she had a mild degree of androgenetic alopecia was being liberal. Clearly, at that point, the most significant contribution to her slight physical problem came from her own mind. Although my preference would have been to refer her for a psychiatric consultation and possible medication, it was clear the time was not yet right. Her dignity was paramount at that point. She needed attention, reassurance, and sympathy for what was, for her, entirely real and very threatening. Sometimes this kind of acceptance from a medical doctor whom the patient trusts is enough to make an obsession recede sufficiently to restore peace of mind.

I wondered whether something might be going on that could be causing her to displace her anxiety in one arena and channel it into this preoccupation, which could be contained in a small, manageable corner of her life.

"Would you say there's any unusual difficulty in your life, Nancy?"

"Only the fact that I'm losing my hair. *That's* difficult. Every woman wants to look her best, but for me it's extra important. You see, my husband is quite an important trial lawyer, and he expects me to do a lot of entertaining. That's fine, because I love parties and people, but if this gets too much worse, I don't know how I'll be able to keep on facing everybody. It really frightens me."

I could see we were going to go around in circles. I would have to work with what she was giving me and bide my time until I had thoroughly gained her trust. Certainly, since she did have a mild androgen excess, it was worth trying some topical treatment and perhaps some low-level hormonal therapy.

"I only asked about anything that might be stressful or difficult in the rest of your life because it could be adding to your physical problem."

"I just don't think so," she replied. "Not at all."

"Well, then, I want to give you a slightly different preparation of Rogaine than the one you've been using. I'm going to add some retinoic acid, which is the active ingredient in Retin-A. We've found that this particular cocktail makes the Rogaine penetrate better. It also increases the blood flow to your scalp, which means more nutrients reach your hair roots."

She nodded happily, clearly pleased that I appeared to have found a treatable condition.

"By the way, does that mean I need to protect my hair from the sun? I know you can't go out in the sun if you're using Retin-A."

"That's a good question, but no. In this case, you're on a low dosage, and your hair is sufficient to protect your scalp. If we decided to increase the dosage at some point, you would need to wear a hat."

"Well, I usually do wear a hat, to cover up my problem. I was just wondering whether I needed to get one of those sunscreens for hair."

"I do want to warn you that hair regrowth is a slow process. It may take six months or more before you'll see an improvement, and frankly, not everyone responds to Rogaine. I want to see you once a month, so I can check your progress and make sure your hair loss isn't getting any worse."

Then I thought of one more step Nancy could take. Its only effect in her case might be that of a placebo, but I wanted to do everything I could think of to reduce her anxiety by making her feel more in control. "Another thing I think might help, Nancy, is to avoid foods that contain androgens, like brewer's yeast, peanut oil, and wheat germ." This advice also holds true in acne, another skin disorder related to androgen excess.

"That's interesting," she said, brightening. "We use quite a lot of peanut oil in Chinese cooking, and I do mix wheat germ into my cereal in the morning. I was always told that it was good for me."

"Wheat germ *is* good for you, but I think in view of your symptoms, it would be best to forgo it for a while. Another thing you can do is wash your hair often—even every day. I know this might seem as if you're stressing it too much, but in fact the sebum—the

oily, waxy stuff that builds up on your scalp—contains androgens.''

"What kind of shampoo should I use, then?''

"The diluted baby shampoo you're already using is fine. If you
find your hair feels dry, you can condition it as often as you need
to. I'm sure you know never to brush it when it's wet, because it's
much more apt to break.''

We shook hands. "Thank you, Dr. Pratt,'' she said. "This is the
first time I've felt hopeful about all this.''

Psychocutaneous diseases, those in which there is an interaction
between the mind and the skin, are traditionally grouped into
three broad categories. First are conditions whose origin is strictly
psychological. These include delusions and hallucinations of skin
infestations, some chronic pain syndromes, repetitive hair pulling
or skin excoriation, and factitious dermatitis, in which patients'
skin problems result from their own, usually unconscious, self-
mutilation. Arthur and I have treated many patients afflicted with
this tragic syndrome.

Charlotte, a college student in her mid-twenties, picks at her
face until it is raw. She can't control it, isn't even aware her own
hands are the perpetrators of her painful and ugly lesions. The last
time I saw her, she told me she had just been in her seventh
wedding. "Always a bridesmaid, never the bride,'' she said with a
rueful little laugh. It saddened me to see this lovely girl who was
quite possibly facing a lifetime of loneliness. For every time she is
invited out, she reopens all her lesions and scabs, rubbing and
picking them until they are bleeding, forcing her to cancel the
date. With her wounds healed, she is a bright and appealing-
looking girl and is asked out often. Accordingly, the cycle is repeated with some frequency. After her remark about being always
a bridesmaid, I decided to introduce my suspicions as to the origin
of her wounds. I knew a direct question would make her defen-
sive, so I wondered aloud whether her sores might possibly be
self-inflicted, albeit unconsciously so, and whether we should perhaps consider adding a psychiatrist to the treatment team. But she
responded with utter mystification. "That can't be true,'' she said
without a trace of defensiveness. "I just keep waking up with

these things!" But while Charlotte herself was merely puzzled by my suggestion, her mother was livid, calling to tell me I had insulted not only her daughter but indeed the whole family. This is a fairly common response on the part of parents of such patients. Many, but by no means all, patients with self-inflicted skin trauma have been the victims of emotional or physical abuse. It was beyond the range of my training to even attempt to explore these issues, but it wouldn't have mattered, because Charlotte's mother refused to let her come back to see me. I often wonder about her. Cases like hers frequently respond to psychotherapy and psychiatric medications. I can only hope Charlotte will find her way to a skillful therapist and that he or she will know a good dermatologist or cosmetic surgeon who can rid her face of its ever-deepening scars.

The second category of mind-skin disease includes conditions with a physical basis that may be triggered or exacerbated by emotional stress. Some cases of hives, severe itching, flushing, and disorders of the sweat glands that produce either foul-smelling body odor or excessive sweating all may fall under this rubric. In these patients it is essential to ascertain that no underlying medical disease might be causing the symptoms. For instance, itching may be the first sign of certain cancers, liver disease, or internal parasites. Unlike patients whose symptoms are psychological in origin, those with these types of mixed symptoms, in which skin problems are obvious to the doctor yet don't respond to standard treatments, are often quite willing to accept that stress or anxiety is contributing to their problem. In fact, they may be relieved to find that nothing is seriously wrong with their skin. Sometimes just learning their skin symptoms aren't serious is enough to make the symptoms recede.

The third group of diseases we commonly encounter are clearly physical, genetic, or environmental in origin but frequently, though not always, worsened by stress. Psoriasis, eczema, and acne may fall into this category. Often, when common skin diseases do not respond well to treatment, it is because the underlying emotional kindling has yet to be exposed.

Because I had once considered psychology as a possible profession, I found the frequent patients with problems involving both mind and skin particularly fascinating. Even though there are three neat categories for classifying these patients, they are somewhat arbitrary. The more we learn about mind-body interactions, the further we depart from the Cartesian duality of mind and body that has probably somewhat hindered our ability to treat our patients, no matter what their complaints. I applaud the new holism in medicine. For if the brain and the rest of the human body aren't a continuum, how else can we explain phenomena like the crucifixation stigmata that appear on the hands and feet of certain extremely devout people at Easter? Or the condition known as *mnemoderma,* or skin memory, in which gentle stroking of an area once afflicted with hives will elicit paroxysmal itching. Or the case quoted in one of the standard dermatology texts of a young soldier in World War II who developed dramatic hair loss four times during his tour of duty in the South Pacific. Each time, it happened within two weeks of his participation in an island invasion. Each time his unit was furloughed, his hair grew in. After the war was over, his hair grew back permanently.

In order to treat Nancy, I had to try to categorize her complaint. I had at least to decide which end of the mind-skin spectrum was most involved and which was the best place to try to break the circuit causing her symptoms.

Although I had begun by thinking Nancy's complaint was almost certainly in the first category of pure psychological symptoms, as time went on, I came to believe she did have true physical symptoms—however mild and insignificant—and that the force of her obsession and her consequent anxiety were exacerbating the mild physical condition. That is the difficult part for me as a doctor, because these patients use their slight physical problems to channel their deeper anxiety. If I can actually treat just the skin symptom without addressing the feelings fueling the problem— and often it's impossible to do so—the patient's emotional symptoms may get far worse. Nancy's preoccupation with her hair was probably classifiable as an increasingly recognized chronic disorder now referred to as *body dysmorphic disorder.* Symptoms of this disorder typically involve the face or head but may involve any other part of the body. Patients with this syndrome usually do have some minimal physical abnormality, which becomes exaggerated in their minds until it comes to dominate their thoughts. For instance, mildly thinning hair like Nancy's, a large nose, or thin lips become the source of tortured thoughts. Some people who are severely afflicted come to believe that others are horrified to see them, when in fact their appearance is entirely normal.

After I had seen Nancy six or seven times and initiated medical treatment, I decided it was time to meet the underlying problem head-on.

"There's another treatment I think we ought to consider, Nancy. Of course," I hastened to interject, "we'll continue the minoxidil. But there have been a number of reports in the literature recently that conditions like yours respond well to low doses of the newer antidepressants, like Prozac and Zoloft, in addition to standard medical therapy. I'm not suggesting you're depressed, but the fascinating thing about these drugs is their ability to treat many different medical problems. For instance, I have a patient who has been tortured because her scalp itches, particularly at night, when she's trying to fall asleep. I started her on Prozac, and for the first time she's had some relief. What do you think? I think it's worth considering."

"Absolutely out of the question," she said quietly. "Antidepressants are for people with mental problems—not for normal people whose hair is falling out. I would be terrified to take drugs like those, and on top of that, I'd be embarrassed to go to the drug store with a prescription for them."

"Many people feel that way, Nancy. The drugs really are nothing to fear. Most people don't even know they're taking them, except that their symptoms disappear. But I respect your decision. I just wanted to give you that option." I knew enough had been said. I was frustrated, because I was almost positive an antidepressant would have helped break the cycle of stress leading to hormonal imbalance, which was contributing to the mild hair loss, which was causing her anxiety to begin with. Perhaps, having planted the seed, I would try to reopen the discussion in the future.

One day soon afterward, Nancy asked me if I believed in alternative therapies. In fact, I feel that the current reconsideration of some of these older forms of healing is one of the most fascinating and encouraging trends in medicine today.

"Yes, I'm open to many of them," I told her. "Did you have anything particular in mind?"

"Well, I read somewhere that homeopathy sometimes cures things when everything else has failed. . . ."

"I don't know much about homeopathy myself," I said, "but I'm sure I could help you find a doctor who works with it. More and more M.D.s are using it and other complementary therapies in addition to conventional medicine."

"Would you ever try something like that if you were me?"

"Sure, I might," I said. "It would depend on what was wrong and who would be treating me."

At that time, I had never experienced firsthand much medicine of any sort. Checkups and prenatal care were about it, so I had never had cause to look for alternative treatments. Recently, however, I had had the unusual experience of being treated by one of my own patients. I had been doing facial peels and electrolysis on Lara for a year or two. I knew she was a nurse at a nearby hospital, but one day she told me she was studying foot reflexology and that she hoped to change careers and open a practice of her own once she was certified. Foot reflexology is a system of healing in which different areas of the foot are thought to be connected to specific organs. Practitioners believe that by massaging areas of the foot corresponding to these organs, they can actually influence the organs' functioning. Although I could imagine such a connection might be physiologically possible, I was still skeptical and surprised at Lara's change of profession.

"What I'm wondering, Dr. Pratt," she said to me one day as I worked on her, "is whether you'll consider letting me work on *you*. I need to treat thirty patients in order to graduate."

I thought about the idea for a day or two and then decided to go ahead and try it. Another of my patients had had her colitis cleared up by shiatsu, and I was intrigued by the apparent power of these forms of healing, even if I couldn't quite see a physical basis for them. I invited Lara to come at the end of the day so that she could work on me in one of my treatment rooms. If nothing else, it would give me a better sense of how comfortable my room was for my patients.

Two hours passed in a dream. At one point, Arthur stuck his

head in the door, apparently to ask me a question, looked alarmed, and quickly retreated. At the end of the session, Lara asked me what I had felt.

"Well, first of all, I felt like I didn't have a care in the world—which was nice. And at one point, when you were working around the ball of my foot, I felt this strong tingling in my neck, which stopped as soon as you moved to another part of my foot."

"One thing I noticed was that you might be a little hypothyroid. You probably ought to get it checked."

"Well," I said, "that's one explanation for my morning tiredness." I made a mental note to have Arthur draw some blood for a thyroid screen.

After Lara left, I went upstairs to see when Arthur was planning to finish for the day. "What was going on in there?" he asked slightly bemused. "Isn't that person a patient of yours?"

"Yes, she's doing a course in foot reflexology and she asked if she could work on me."

"It's not a specialty I'm familiar with," he said, and began to gather up the things on his desk.

"Neither am I, but I thought it would be interesting, and it was. She thinks I might be borderline hypothyroid."

He nodded wearily as if to placate me before I did something even weirder.

My thyroid turned out to be normal, and although I have no way of objectively assessing the therapeutic worth of foot reflexology, it certainly felt good, and I continue to be intrigued by it and other therapies that are becoming increasingly mainstream. In my mind, an alliance between modern Western medical technology and knowledge and some of the more ancient modalities may add some synergy to our armamentarium. For example, I was fascinated recently to read about some studies in Germany in which oncologists are injecting minute amounts of cancer chemotherapeutic drugs directly into the appropriate acupuncture meridians and then stimulating the meridians with a low electric current, rather than blasting the whole patient with near-killing doses of these toxic drugs. To me, such innovative therapies are intriguing, and we owe it to our patients to learn all we can about such healing techniques.

I continued to see Nancy Cheng at frequent intervals over the next year. When she felt that the minoxidil–retinoic acid combination was not helping stave off her hair loss, we discontinued it.

We began to discuss the possibility of some hormonal manipulations to lower her androgen levels.

"My suggestion is that we start you on birth control pills with high estrogen and a nonandrogenic progesterone. . . ."

"No. I cannot take those," she said, pushing the heels of her hands against my desk. "Early on, my gynecologist suggested I might be able to control my hair loss that way, so I agreed to try, but I started to get so bloated and fat that I couldn't fit into my clothes. You can see I haven't been able to get rid of that last ten pounds."

In fact, Nancy was extremely thin. A loss of ten pounds would have left her clothes hanging like laundry from her frame.

"We could try a blood pressure drug called spironolactone. The only thing about that is that you would have to come in pretty regularly, so I could monitor your potassium level."

"I just hate all these intrusions into my body. Hormones scare me. I'm always reading about the pill causing breast cancer and strokes, and I've tried to avoid things like that. I don't mind things you put *on* my body, but I'm very wary about putting things into it."

"Then why don't we see whether a progesterone solution you can apply to your scalp will help."

Unfortunately, the progesterone solution did not help. Neither Nancy nor I could see a change in her hair pattern after seven months of treatment. I suggested she consider some of the other hormonal treatments I had outlined for her, but again she rejected them all.

At one point, she asked me about hair transplantation.

"I have no wish to make my problem more obvious," she said. "Nor do I wish to go around looking like Senator Proxmire, with all those ugly plugs sticking out of his scalp, but I heard that Dr. Balin performs hair transplantation by a single hair technique. Would that help me?"

"The new technique, using micrografts, is much better, much more effective, and certainly much more subtle. We make a minute incision with a needle and then insert one or two of your own hairs harvested from the back of your head. Most, but not all, take and grow very naturally."

This is an operation some of our male patients request from time to time. Even a man who is quite bald can benefit from the insertion of several hundred hairs, even if they do not restore a thick head of hair, because they frame his face in a more flattering manner. Patients are often astonished how much better they look with just this subtle replacement.

"Well," Nancy said, "I hoped it might help."

About a year and a half into Nancy's treatment, Arthur and I attended a meeting of the Society of Investigative Dermatology in Atlanta. There we heard a presentation by a dermatologist from New York who had developed a progesterone formulation he injected directly into the scalp.

When I told her about this approach, Nancy was interested in seeing this doctor, who had great expertise in treating hair loss in women. "I don't want you to think I'm abandoning you," she said after I had told her about the presentation, "but maybe I should go see him, just in case those shots can cure my problem. Will you and he be able to work together if he does change my treatment?"

"Of course. Doctors often work in collaboration. At this point, I'd be interested in hearing his assessment. He's a world-famous specialist in this area, and I thought his treatment ideas sounded promising. By all means, go see him. I spoke to him briefly at the meeting about your case. I can call him and arrange to have your chart sent up there."

After seeing her and repeating the blood tests, the other physician agreed Nancy's hair loss was indeed due to a mild degree of androgen excess and would probably never become noticeably worse. However, since Nancy clearly wanted to try the progesterone injections, he saw no reason not to proceed. He had given her the first injections in New York and sent her home with a supply of the formulation, which I would inject in Nancy's scalp—on the crown and around her temples—once a month.

Despite the pain and expense of the injections, Nancy felt they were doing some good. I did not see any change. Objectively, Nancy had lost perhaps three percent of her hair over the two years I had followed her, an amount not atypical for a woman her age. Most women would not have perceived this level of thinning.

After I had been seeing Nancy for nearly three years, I began to notice that the hair at her temples was receding, albeit at a slow rate. Certainly it had not reached an abnormal level, but her pattern of hair thinning was more typical of a woman at least ten years older.

At that time, Arthur and I were beginning to be interested in an adrenal hormone called DHEA and its role in the aging process. As we age, levels of both testosterone and its precursor, DHEA, begin to decline. By age eighty, one produces only 10–20 percent of the DHEA a normal teenager would produce. Several research groups were finding that DHEA might be a useful marker of biologic age and longevity potential. Others were finding it could enhance the function of the immune system by stimulating certain types of white blood cells and that it could increase the life span of laboratory animals by 50 percent. However, it was not these fascinating but unconventional roles for DHEA that interested me for Nancy. Rather, it was DHEA's physiologic role as a precursor to many other hormones.

Like many problems in endocrinology, a diagram of the pathways that theoretically were coming into play in this case would be a series of interconnected loops, circles, and switchbacks. With Nancy's hair loss actually beginning to be apparent to me, I wondered whether it might be symptomatic of premature aging. When I had her blood tested, I found her DHEA level was indeed low. Since DHEA is a precursor to many other hormones, it may also act as a reservoir to pump up those whose levels were tapering. Perhaps her low level of DHEA was influencing her poor hair growth. Supplementing it was an experimental approach, but one I felt was justified in this difficult case.

Although Nancy had earlier rejected the idea of taking hormones, she was intrigued enough about DHEA and its potential anti-aging and antiobesity effects that she wanted to try it, although she was aware its potential effect on her condition was theoretical only.

I was rather optimistic about my theory. Besides the possibility of DHEA's increasing the levels of various hormonal precursors, I had also thought of another pathway by which it might stop Nancy's hair loss. Feeling quite pleased with what I thought was an innovative solution and one that might end up working for other patients, I presented it to Arthur over the dinner table.

He listened politely, with no discernible expression on his face until I had finished. He said nothing for about sixty seconds. Many people find Arthur's silences intimidating, but I knew that it just meant he was computing. Well, good news, I thought. My idea was so clever it wasn't totally obvious. Arthur was having to think about it for a minute. As his silence continued, I was just waiting for him to burst out with some version of "Eureka!" My mind began to design a study protocol. I could already see our paper featured in one of the better journals—maybe even the *New England Journal of Medicine. . . .*

"Loretta," Arthur finally said. "I don't know how you thought this up."

I could feel a glow of pride creeping across my face, but then I noticed his expression. It contained nothing of the anticipated Eureka response.

"This is just Lamarckian. If this kind of reasoning were true, then you could cut the legs off a mother frog and all her babies would be born without legs." (Lamarck was an eighteenth-century scientist who believed acquired characteristics were inheritable.)

"Let me make sure I understand: you're saying that by giving *more* androgens in the form of DHEA, you're increasing the levels of androgen-binding globulin, which will bind to the already excessive androgens and inactivate them?"

"Well, yes," I said, hesitantly. It wasn't easy arguing with Arthur. He could retreat into his enormous mental library and come up with studies to support anything he thought was true. "I think it makes sense," I added defiantly.

Arthur shook his head in wonderment. "Well, it could be worth a try, but not for that reason," he said.

"It makes perfect sense," I attempted. "Anyway, forget the androgen-binding globulin. That's just an alternate pathway I thought of. The other possibility is that she's just aging prematurely and not making enough female hormones to offset the androgens. She can't tolerate birth control pills, which would obviously be my first choice, so DHEA as a precursor to those same hormones might be just the ticket."

"Oh, what a tangled web you weave," Arthur sighed.

"Well, I think it's worth a try, and so does my patient. Maybe I've made a major discovery that I'll become famous for and you'll have pooh-poohed it," I said, laughing.

Arthur shrugged and went back to his dinner. "Better monitor the DHEA levels well, so you can document what the drug does for her."

His vote of no confidence didn't leave me feeling entirely sanguine, but my theory *still* made sense to me. DHEA is a safe way of manipulating the relevant hormones, and plenty of studies were coming out showing its multitude of anti-aging benefits. Arthur himself was beginning to explore its use as part of a life-extension regimen. Even if it didn't benefit Nancy's hair as I hoped it would, it might make her feel better. New studies were showing it controlled depression, and since I believed her problem to be depression as much as anything else, that was another point in favor of my approach. I decided to do a computer search and put in calls to a couple of the authors of recent papers on DHEA.

A week or two after Arthur's and my discussion, Nancy appeared in my office for her monthly scalp injection looking much more cheerful than usual.

"Notice anything different?" she asked.

Clearly, she expected me to. But just as I was unable to observe her alopecia through quite the same lens as she, on that day it was equally difficult to appreciate whatever change she had in mind.

"It's a bit hard to tell," I said as noncommittally as possible. "But your hair looks fuller, somehow."

"It sure is!" she chortled. And then she removed five or six hairpins from her head and lifted a sort of toupee from her crown.

"A hairdresser friend of mine made this from all the hair I've lost over the past couple of years." She pushed it across the desk toward me. It was a skillful piece of handiwork.

"What a good idea," was all I could think of to say.

"I think so. Don't feel that I'm not grateful for all you've done. Without your treatments I'd be as bald as a billiard, but this hides those hideous areas of scalp, so I can at least face the rest of the world without wearing a hat every minute of the day. I'm going to keep collecting all my hair, so that when the time comes, my friend can make me a more extensive hairpiece to cover my whole scalp."

Nancy still comes in every month for her progesterone shots and has recently begun to take DHEA. She still worries that everyone is repelled by her balding scalp, but her alliance with her hairdresser has proved to be therapeutic. Together they devise becoming new hairstyles that use the hairpiece and, best of all in her mind, serve to cover up her "problem."

Although I might have wished Nancy had allowed me to try a psychopharmacologic approach, which might have permitted her a far greater degree of comfort early on, she chose her own path. As time has passed, it has become apparent she is losing hair at a rate slightly accelerated for her age. I would say her symptoms lie somewhere on the mysterious cusp between the mind and the body. While, regrettably, she is still tortured by her dread of someday being entirely bald, she has been able to relax in the knowledge that few besides her hairdresser will know for sure.

Ethel Tuck and Ernestina, her middle-aged daughter, could have stepped from the pages of a textbook on psychocutaneous diseases. Our first encounter with them began literally with a bang.

I was just finishing up electrodessicating some red spider veins on the nose and cheeks of a middle-aged actor when suddenly there was a loud crash from the parking lot. This was followed by a single blast from a car's horn, then silence. Thankfully, I had just put down the electric needle and was examining the actor's face through a magnifier. I peered through the slats of the venetian blind, but my view of the parking lot was blocked by the prow of a large blue-and-white car in the parking space just outside my window.

I had recently joined Arthur's practice in Pennsylvania. Arthur was away, fulfilling the rigorous training for certification in Mohs surgery, which meant that he spent Monday through Friday at Baylor Medical Center in Dallas. I hoped there hadn't been an accident in the parking lot. I had all my caseload and some of Arthur's patients as well. I could certainly live without any nonmedical logistical problems to deal with in his absence.

I called into the reception room, "Pam, would you go out there and see what's going on?"

She returned a few minutes later. "No problem," she said, raising her eyebrows high. "That was your five o'clock patient, Ethel Tuck. She was just trying to park her car. She's fine, the building's fine, and her car's no worse than it was."

I looked at my watch. I decided to use the five minutes between the actor and the patient in the parking lot to return some phone calls and go over the typed reports on some of the morning's patients. By ten after five, I began to wonder what had become of my patient. Just as I got up to send Pam out to look for her, an obese woman who looked to be about fifty appeared in the doorway.

She jerked her thumb behind her. "She be coming in a minute," she said. "She's just getting her things."

This exact scenario, from the collision on arrival to the twenty-minute delay before she could extricate herself from the car and get into the office, was to be repeated nearly every time Ethel Tuck came. The office staff were so afraid she was going to ram their cars in her wild maneuverings that they began to park in a vacant lot across the street on days she had an appointment.

I stood in the doorway of the office. "Come right in, Mrs. Tuck," I said. "Your friend can have a seat here in the waiting room."

"Oh no, she's not my friend. She's my daughter!" Mrs. Tuck crowed, clearly tickled at her joke. "Can't she come in while you talk to me? I have to keep an eye on her." She dropped her voice and tapped her forehead. "She ain't right in the head."

We all crowded into my office. They were both built like Botero giantesses, and their combined mass seemed out of scale in the small room.

Ethel Tuck hadn't filled out a medical questionnaire, so I gave her a form and asked her to complete it. I sat at my desk opposite them and busied myself with the day's charts. When she had finished, she passed it to me. She was seventy-eight years old, but like so many African-Americans, her unlined skin alone would have been an unreliable clue to her true age, which was more accurately discernible from her stooped posture and arthritic gait.

Ethel Tuck had medical problems typical of her age group—high blood pressure and adult onset diabetes. But what brought her to me was by far the worst of her problems, she felt.

"I got the scabies," she said, leaning across the desk to deliver this pronouncement in a stage whisper.

Scabies is a contagious skin disease caused by *Sarcoptes scabiei,* the itch mite, a microscopic creature that has found food and lodging in the human skin since biblical times. In 1099, Saint Hildegard wrote in her treatise *Physika* that scabies was due to a small insect she called "snebelza." While the cause of scabies was clear to the laity for centuries, most physicians were not yet ready to accept the concept of infectious vectors of disease until the mid-nineteenth century when the connection between the mites and the misery they caused was at last generally accepted.

Scabies mites are denizens of the warm, protected areas between the fingers and toes, the armpits, genitals, nipples, and navel, but they also seem to enjoy life on the wrists, elbows, and ankles. Once they have invaded, they burrow their way into the underside of the epidermis, dropping eggs as they go. As the epidermis proceeds on its monthly life cycle, older mite tunnels are pushed to the surface, the horny layer on top flakes off, liberating a generation of immature mites, and new passages are formed beneath, so that the mites' cycle can continue.

The human host can be literally maddened by the itching. As Ethel Tuck described to me the familiar tortures inflicted on her by these mites, she became animated and histrionic.

"What are your symptoms like?" I asked her.

"I scratch and they bite, and I scratch and they crawl around under my skin and bite me in another place. I scratch all night long, just like a dog!" she shouted, suddenly jumping to her feet to lean across the desk at me. (In fact, a related mite causes the canine condition known as sarcoptic mange, in which a dog can literally denude itself in a frenzy of scratching and licking.)

"How long have you had this problem, Mrs. Tuck?"

She sat back down. "I've had them for years and years. And I can tell you when I got them."

"When do you think it was?"

"I got them a long time ago, from a dirty man. Oh, he was a

dirty man! He put them nasty things inside my body, and they traveled into my system, and they came out through my feet. And I ain't never gotten rid of them. Never."

She began to fumble in her capacious purse. "Wait a minute, wait a minute. Here!" she said, passing a small box across my desk. In the bottom were some particles she said were "nits" that she had scraped from her toes.

The matchbox sign! This is a behavior so typical of patients with delusions of parasitosis that it is almost diagnostic in and of itself. Sometimes patients will go to extremes to bring in samples of their tormentors. We have had patients who prepared labeled, mounted slide displays that would have done a graduate microbiologist proud. But even though Ethel's entire demeanor, especially in combination with the matchbox sign, suggested she was delusional, several possibilities had to be considered after I had had a chance to examine her.

With Ernestina in attendance in my examining room, I went carefully over Ethel Tuck's body, but I found nothing remarkable beyond some mild dandruff. Until I reached her feet, which looked like the victims of some barbaric torture. Both were so hot and swollen that I was amazed she had been able to stand, encasing them in the tightly laced saddle shoes she had worn. They were clearly infected and even had signs of cellulitis, meaning that the infection had spread down to the deepest layer of the skin, the subcutaneous. But the typical scabies burrows, often with mites visible in them, were not to be seen.

"You see that!" she cried as I got to her toes. "Them scabies bit so hard, I had to dig them out with a razor."

"You did *what*?"

"I took a razor blade to them and cut them out of my toes, but they got right back in there. But I heard you can give me some kind of medicine that will make them go away."

"Mrs. Tuck," I said, "cutting your toes with a razor blade is not the way to get rid of scabies. Now, I want you to promise me you'll never do that again."

"Then you got to give me some medicine to make them stop bugging me." Again, she laughed uproariously at her pun.

Nothing suggested she had any real infestation, but before I wrote off her symptoms to a delusion, I knew I must make certain her odd behavior and work with the razor blade weren't causing me to overlook a deeper medical diagnosis. I mentally scrolled through the list of possibilities. People with certain neurologic disorders, such as multiple sclerosis, frequently have what are called paresthesias, or abnormal feelings in the skin, often described as crawling and biting sensations. But usually these patients don't appear frantic and delusional. Ethel had stated on her history that she had once had a venereal disease, so it was always possible her symptoms were due to neurosyphilis, or syphilis of the central nervous system, whose victims may suffer delusions of parasitosis. People with organic brain syndromes, like Alzheimer's disease, could have such symptoms, but Ethel didn't fit the picture of the typical Alzheimer's patient, even an early-stage one. Often, long-term users of amphetamine and cocaine act quite psychotic, and it is not uncommon for them to have formication, the sensation of small creatures crawling on their skin. People addicted to heroin and synthetic opiates like Demerol are often plagued by itching, but it is most often around the face. Ethel had no tracks from injecting drugs, and she didn't have the jumpy, sweaty, paranoid presence or runny nose emblematic of people who snort large amounts of cocaine and amphetamine.

I remembered the words of one of my teachers, who had started his career as a psychiatrist and then become a dermatologist. "In such cases, Loretta, you have to let these people know you're on their side and that you believe they do have a problem that's driving them nuts. Chances are they've been from doctor to doctor and their reception at various offices has not left them feeling very good about themselves. Since most of them are already depressed to begin with, you have to be their friend first in order to help them as a physician."

My personal standard of care has always been to treat my patients, even the difficult ones, even those with whom I could not empathize at all, like members of my own family. This goes back to an incident that occurred before I had even fully made up my mind to go to medical school.

My mother and I had taken my father to the emergency room, because he had fallen down and hurt his ankle. My father had a drinking problem, but he was the kindest of fathers and husbands, and his drinking never turned mean. He was more apt to fall asleep at the wrong moment or, as he had on this occasion, to fall down and hurt himself. Even then I knew that triage was the order of the day in any emergency room and that such problems as gunshot wounds, heart attacks, and severe stomach pain had to be attended to first. But on this late weekday afternoon, the ER seemed relatively quiet. (As a med student, I would come to understand that this midafternoon lull was typical of the ER. For some reason, most heart attack patients come in either in the morning or late at night, while the violent injuries related to drinking and drugs usually come later in the evening.) After all the patients who had been waiting when we walked in had been seen, and even a few walk-ins who didn't seem seriously afflicted were also ushered in first, my mother, quite reasonably, became upset. Leaving me to watch my father, she walked over to the nurses' station, where a resident was eating a sandwich and reading a journal.

"Are you in charge here?" I heard her ask.

"I'm eating my dinner," he replied with astonishing rudeness.

"I don't understand why my husband has been kept waiting so long. He is ill and in pain. Why can't somebody take care of him?"

"What's the hurry?" the young doctor answered with a shrug. "He's done this to himself."

I glanced at my father, hoping he hadn't heard. But I could tell by the way he hung his head and stared at his shoes that he had. I've never forgotten that incident. It has made for my own Golden Rule of patient care.

First, I had to gain Ethel's trust, and the way to do that was by treating what I could and taking the rest of her complaints seriously without, at the same time, reinforcing her delusion. I decided to begin by treating the infection and cellulitis and examining her matchbox exhibit under the microscope. There was always the possibility that she really did have some type of parasite—if not mites, perhaps lice or bedbugs.

I took a sample of the fluid oozing from her two large toes, so that the lab could determine what type of bacterium was causing the infection and which antibiotic would be most effective against it. I also gave her a prescription for an ointment to apply to her toes and a solution in which to soak her feet several times a day.

She promised to call me in two days, when I would have the results of her cultures and could choose the right antibiotic.

Two days later, after the sensitivity testing had been done, I left an antibiotic prescription for her at the reception desk with a message that I wanted to see her again in three weeks, after she had taken all the pills. When she and Ernestina arrived, they came on foot, but they initiated another ritual they were to maintain at every appointment thereafter. First Ernestina, and then Ethel, went into the bathroom and stayed there for about fifteen minutes, the water running at full-bore the entire time. Then they double-checked the time of the next appointment and left.

On the next visit, Ethel's big toes were even more swollen and infected.

"Ethel," I said sternly, looking her in the eye, "have you been cutting your skin with a razor blade again?"

"No, ma'am, Dr. Pratt," she said, looking right back at me.

"But Ethel, it certainly looks like you have. Look here at your left foot. You've sliced the nail right off your big toe."

"No, Dr. Pratt, the scabies did that. But I think I got them under control now for sure."

"Why is that?"

"Yesterday, when the exterminator came to my building, I got him to spray some kind of special stuff to kill those scabies. I made him spray my bedroom and Ernestina's, and then I took all our sheets and I threw them in the garbage pail, and Ernestina took out the garbage and walked ten blocks before she dumped it."

Her blood test had come back negative for neurosyphilis, and I was sure she was not experiencing the paresthesias of a neurologic disease. She seemed a classic example of a person with delusions of parasitosis, or *Ekbom syndrome.* This is different from the type of global delusional behavior one might see in a schizophrenic, in that her belief she was harboring "scabies" was her only symptom. In the rest of her life, she appeared to function well, even logically. She could drive a car, she had worked as a nanny for many years and was still in touch with her former charges and their families, and she had gotten help for Ernestina, who seemed fond of her in a bemused but tolerant way. Even the steps she had taken to eradicate the invaders—trying to cut them out of her foot with a razor blade and trying to rid her home of them—had a certain logic. Moreover, it was entirely possible she *had* some sort of parasitic infestation at one point and that the delusion had built from there.

"Ethel," I said gently, "you are hurting yourself by using that razor blade on your feet. You are getting a very bad infection. I want to help you, but I can't continue to treat you if you're going to keep hurting yourself."

"But those nits are driving me *crazy*," she wailed. "I can't sleep at night till they go to sleep and leave me alone. And I never know when they're going to go to sleep, 'cause it depends on what I eat."

"I looked at what you brought me in that matchbox, and I didn't see the type of mite that causes scabies or any other type of bug. But if you see any others, bring them next week and I'll look at them again. In the meantime, I want you to keep soaking your feet, applying the ointment I gave you, and taking the pills. But above all, you have to stop picking."

"You see!" Ernestina said. But her mother ignored her.

At Ethel's next appointment, I was pleased to note that her toes looked better.

"I don't think those scabies like those pills," she said. "I can still feel them in there, but they don't move around as much."

I again took a culture and told her I would call her to tell her whether she needed to continue the antibiotics.

"You mean you're going to take my medicine away?" she shrieked so loudly that I pushed the office door shut. "You mean to tell me that?"

"Ethel, the pills made your feet feel better because they helped heal the infection you caused with the razor blade. It's not good for you to take antibiotics when you don't need them."

"But I do need them," she shouted, leaning across my desk.

"Ethel, they won't help what you have. I don't think your problems are being caused by mites, but even if you did have them, these pills would not get rid of them. That's not what they're for," I said firmly. "I will not give them to you if you do not need them."

"I'm telling you I need them. If those scabies come back like they was, I'm going to cut my foot right off!" she shouted even louder. Pam stuck her head in the door to see if everything was all right. I wished Arthur were there or that I could muster the same soft-spoken but no-nonsense manner with which he handled difficult patients.

I stood up. "Mrs. Tuck, I have given you my medical opinion. I am going to have to ask you to leave this office. I cannot continue to treat people who are argumentative and disruptive to the other patients."

She dropped back down in her chair and burst into tears. "No, please, *please* don't send me away. Please, Dr. Pratt, you're the only doctor who has ever helped me," she sobbed. Ernestina nodded sorrowfully in agreement.

"Then you will have to promise to follow my medical advice and never to raise your voice in this office again."

"Yes, ma'am, Dr. Pratt," she said contritely, wiping the tears from her cheeks.

"Now, I want to see you in one week. I did not find anything on your skin today that might be causing your symptoms, but I understand how much your feet are bothering you. The ointment and the soaks will make them feel better." I wanted to see whether her symptoms might resolve once the infection was completely cleared up. There was a chance they would, although I was doubtful.

I called her during the week and told her she would not need to keep taking the antibiotics, and she accepted my instructions without argument. But when she and Ernestina arrived for her next appointment, she was once again very upset.

"I knew they'd come back when I stopped taking the medicine. And now they've invaded my whole system. Look in here." She handed me a glass jar filled with small, dark particles. "That's B.M.," she explained. "You can see them in there. And now I think they're getting into Ernestina."

I did not want Ethel's problem to segue into a *folie à deux,* which is common in families when one person has an overwhelming delusion. I decided the time had come to try another tack. Psychiatric drugs are often helpful in Ekbom syndrome. My first choice was a drug called pimozide, used in the same types of patients who are treated with Haldol and Thorazine. Although approved in this country only for use in Tourette's syndrome, a neurologic disease, it is also used widely and successfully to treat monosymptomatic delusions like Ethel's. (It has also been used to help patients suffering from pathologic jealousy.)

I checked Ethel's chart. She had no history of the type of heart disease that would rule out the use of pimozide. To be certain, I also ran an EKG, which was normal.

"Ethel, there may be a couple of explanations for your symptoms. I think it's possible you did have scabies at some point, but you don't have it at the moment. Even so, the feelings in your skin can persist. I have treated a couple of other people with the same problem, and I've been able to help them get over all those crawling and biting feelings with a drug called pimozide. Would you like to try it?"

"I'll try anything that will make those bugs leave me alone."

Some might consider it less than open and honest not to level with patients like Ethel and Nancy and tell them that their problem is, to a greater or lesser degree, imaginary. But when it is the mind—not the body—that must be treated, a more diffuse approach is often required. I believe it is a situation in which the end justifies such means—another way of expressing what is called in medicine the risk-benefit ratio. In Nancy's case, I knew she would read the prescription, so I had to tell her in greater detail the drugs I wanted to try, and why. In Ethel's case, the desirable end was surcease from the delusions and an end to her tortured wanderings from doctor to doctor. I knew I could be more vague, because she wanted to be rid of her "infestation" in any way she could. I knew I had a real chance of helping her. I hoped the results would speak for themselves.

Over time, they did. When Ethel returned in two weeks, her main interest was in having me treat the tenderness and residual infection remaining from her razor blade surgery. It was clear she hadn't been cutting herself recently.

"I think the pills are working," Ernestina whispered to me while her mother was in the bathroom. "She's not talking about those scabies and the dirty man who gave them to her all day long, and she's not trying to tell me I've got them when I know I don't." I wondered for a moment how it had come to pass that Ernestina was labeled "not right in the head" when clearly her reality testing—on this issue at least—was far superior to that of her mother.

Five weeks into her treatment, Ethel agreed that the scabies was gone, but she maintained it was only thanks to the new medicine.

I agreed with her, because, in a way, it was true.

Turning Back the Clock

"When I look good, I feel good, and when I feel good, I play good."

WALT FRAZIER,
NEW YORK KNICKS GUARD, 1973

"So, Arthur, your father tells me you did a facelift for him. Didn't you find it a bit unnerving to operate on your own father's face?" queried Rose Bauer, one of my parents' friends.

"Not to mention Oedipal," added her husband, Martin, a psychiatrist of the old school.

We were standing in the food line at a fiftieth-anniversary party honoring another pair of my parents' friends.

"You certainly did a beautiful job," Rose went on. "I can't see a mark, and he looks . . . I don't know—age appropriate. It's as if you lifted some of the years from his face without taking away the person we know. I wish you'd do one for me!"

"It wasn't really a facelift," I said to Rose. "I just tightened his jawline a little."

"Didn't it bother you just a little working on your dad?" Rose insisted.

"I should think that, unconsciously at least, you would resist doing something that would make your father look younger," her husband added. "I don't think I'd want one of my children operating on me—slip of the tongue, slip of the pen, slip of the scalpel—all those parapraxes!"

I remembered that my father had said, "I feel like a forty-year-old. Why should I want to look any older than I feel? *You're* not going to have this problem when you're my age, because you stayed out of the sun. But I didn't, and now I have a chance to look in the mirror and at least recognize what I see."

Another person joined our conversation at this point. "Sometimes I think all this cosmetic surgery is wrong," she said. "I mean, should we all want to look like Audrey Hepburn or Cary Grant, even if we could? Not that plastic surgeons can make that happen *quite* yet. But then, of course, I look at these lines that are beginning to show up on my face, and I look at the slack skin around my jaw, and I wonder how long I'm going to feel that way." The speaker was a studious-looking woman I guessed to be somewhere in her mid-forties.

"Oh, I'm all for plastic surgery," Rose said. "I was just curious about what it must be like to operate on one's own father."

"I suppose attitudes are changing," her husband said. "When I was doing my training, the general feeling was that people who wanted to change their appearance were narcissistic and neurotic, or worse, and that people who wanted plastic surgery for anything except the repair of serious injuries would probably end up even crazier after they could no longer blame their dysfunction on their appearance."

I thought about the human quest for beauty, the changing images of the beautiful, and the increasing power of medicine to perfect human appearance. *Were* the collagen injections, the liposuction, the laser resurfacing, the eyelid and nose jobs causing too much emphasis on the perfection of the surface at the expense of the soul? From time to time people have asked me whether I ever worried I was using my medical knowledge frivolously when I spent time doing cosmetic procedures instead of treating skin diseases. The answer is no. I have always believed that these cosmetic transformations, both minor and radical, work a subtle healing magic of their own. I have seen it happen so many times.

When Loretta and I drifted onto this topic later that evening, she reminded me that Dr. Ivo Pitanguy, the famous Brazilian plastic surgeon, made up his mind to dedicate his surgical skills to the restoration and creation of beauty when a young man whose face he had repaired as best he could following a drastic fire looked at the result in the mirror after the bandages were removed and announced, "I'd rather be dead."

"I wish I had been in on that conversation this afternoon," Loretta said. (Loretta regularly encourages her mother to have a laser skin resurfacing, but although her mother uses Retin-A and some of the other topical treatments we offer, she says she is not yet ready for laser treatment. Like her daughter, Mrs. Pratt is a striking woman with the bone structure of a top model, and she is content in her changing skin. Loretta, for her part, would be happy to restore some of her mother's youthful appearance. "I don't think I'd be falsifying my mother," she always says. "I'd be getting back my mother as I remembered her—before the sun damage and the aging changes started to show.")

"Think of the patients we've had whose lives literally turned around after the removal of a prominent birthmark or a big scar," Loretta said. "I think that just as inner changes can transform a person's outward appearance, the reverse also can be true. To give back some of the lost years or to change a feature or repair a scar can change a patient's life in so many unexpected ways. I'm always fascinated to see what happens. So many of them change course completely. Think of Anne Barker."

Anne Barker visited me first when she was in her mid-forties. At her first appointment, she brought a shopping bag full of skin treatment products and a high school graduation photograph.

"I want to go back to looking more like this," she said, handing me the photograph. "And *these* aren't helping." She lifted up the shopping bag and let it fall to the floor with a clatter.

Normally, I might consider the photograph a bad sign. Loretta and I both agree on the importance of making sure patients have realistic expectations and understand the risks of cosmetic surgery. We feel it is essential to listen as carefully to the patient's unspoken desires as to his or her stated requests. If a woman believes that a blepharoplasty to correct her sagging eyelids or dermabrasion or laser treatment to remove her wrinkles will fundamentally change her life, we are wary. One plastic surgeon wrote in his textbook about a woman who, upon seeing her lifted face for the first time after the bandages were removed, peered into the mirror she was handed and said, "So where's Elizabeth Taylor?" This is a dangerous situation both for the patient and for us. If a man thinks abdominal liposuction and hair implants will automatically give him the sex life of Warren Beatty, we will decline to treat him. We include cosmetic work in our practice because we believe ardently in the importance of people's being comfortable and confident in their physical presentation to the world and in our ability to help our patients achieve this important goal. But there are limits to the magic we can work, and we do everything we can to make this clear at the beginning of our relationship with a new patient. Nevertheless, in many instances, we have seen cosmetic surgery change a patient's entire outlook in a short time. Anne was one of them.

What struck me most about Anne Barker at that first meeting was not that she looked a great deal older than she had in her high school graduation picture, because she didn't. What was striking was the loss of vitality in the figure now before me. In the process of taking her history, I learned why. Anne had married while she was in college and had had a son soon thereafter. The marriage had foundered, and Anne had raised her son, Tommy, by herself. Tommy's great interest in life was science, and his dream was to become a doctor. As a seventeen-year-old, he had joined the local volunteer ambulance squad as an emergency medical technician. Late one night, just after he had graduated from high school, he was called out to a bad car accident. One of the five victims was already dead at the scene, two were relatively unscathed and could be treated at a local hospital, but two of the patients required immediate transport to a university hospital fifty miles away with both a trauma and a burn center. An emergency medical helicopter was dispatched to the scene. Tommy Barker was well trained and experienced for his age, but it was late at night, and accident scenes can be disorienting and chaotic even for experienced emergency workers. For just one second, Tommy forgot a crucial detail from his training, but it was a detail that would have saved his life. Helicopters have two rotors, one on top twelve feet above the ground, and one on the tail, which barely clears the ground by six feet. It is drilled into anyone who works around them that the tail rotor must be considered a rotating guillotine. But that night, as always, Tommy wanted to do his best for the patient. He wanted to make sure the flight nurse aboard the helicopter was aware that even though the driver's burns and head injuries were the most obvious, the steering wheel had been pushed back half a foot, suggesting he could also have sustained an invisible injury of equal magnitude to his heart or abdominal organs. In returning from the wrecked car to the helicopter, eighteen-year-old Tommy Barker forgot about the lethal rear rotor.

Anne, in her grief, became a recluse. She sold her house, moved in with her mother, and mourned for nearly five years.

"Finally, I decided it was time to get back into life. I had been a kindergarten teacher, but I went out and got a real estate license. I started to date, but without much enthusiasm. My son had been my whole life."

One morning, Anne had looked at herself in the mirror and realized that the face she saw there was becoming unfamiliar. Gone was its former velvety texture, gone the peachlike skin tone. Her complexion struck her as lifeless and sallow. For the first time, she noticed a trench between her eyebrows. Smoking, which had been her only solace, had laid a reticulum of fine lines on her upper lip, and she had gained twenty-five pounds, most of which had settled on her hips and thighs. "Suddenly I wondered where my youth had gone. I was in my late thirties when I lost Tommy, and I woke up to find that so much time had just slipped by, I hardly felt I knew the person in the mirror. I just looked tired. I knew I had to do something."

Anne began her transformation by signing up at a Philadelphia salon for a series of facials, but because nothing long-lasting can be achieved by the creams, masks, and surface peels available to beauticians, Anne was disappointed in the results. She stopped smoking and went on a diet, losing most of the weight except for a stubborn pair of saddlebags on her thighs. Still she was not satisfied. If sixty-five-year-old friends of her mother's were able to regain some of their youthful appearance, why couldn't she at age forty-five? One day, she saw an article in the *New York Times* that quoted me. She noted I was in her area and took down my name. After hesitating for several months, she finally pushed herself to make an appointment to see what could be done.

"So here I am," she announced. "I just want to pick up the pieces."

"I can help you turn back the clock somewhat," I replied, "but I can't guarantee that you'll look like the girl in this picture."

"Oh, I know *that*," she said. "I just wanted you to see that I didn't always look like this."

"Good, because we have to be realistic. You're lucky, in that you have some sun damage but not a lot. You have a few fine lines, and you have some uneven pigmentation."

"So all those years of moping indoors were good for something."

"The smoking *has* taken its toll, but we can fix the lines on your upper lip and also the furrow between your eyebrows if you want."

"What about all the fat around my hips and thighs?" she asked. "I saw in your brochure that you do liposuction. I might be interested in that at some point, too."

"You do understand that your medical insurance won't pay for any procedures they don't consider medically necessary."

"Yes, I know. But I've been living pretty frugally. I've hardly spent any of the money I had put aside for Tommy's future, so I might as well invest it in my own future at this point."

Together, Anne and I designed a plan that would work for her—addressing only those features she wished to change and using only techniques with which she felt comfortable. This is one of the parts of my job I enjoy most. There is so much we can do now and so much more on the horizon that it is a great joy to sit with patients and plan how to give them the appearance they've always dreamed of. So much is possible now. I see this work as complementary to my aging research. In my dermatology practice, I can buy time for aging, damaged skin. In my research, I am hoping to learn how we might someday slow, or even prevent, the aging of the human body.

I explained to Anne several approaches that could erase the fine lines on her upper lip and improve the sallowness and uneven color of her complexion. Various types of alpha hydroxy acids (AHAs) can be used to smooth the skin surface, including lactic acid, found in sour milk and tomato juice; citric acid, from citrus fruits; and glycolic acid, from sugar cane juice. Weak solutions of some of these AHAs were at that time beginning to be added with great fanfare to skin care products sold to the general public.

While these formulations are mildly effective in clarifying the skin, they're too weak to do much more. The small contribution they make can gradually become noticeable to the user over many months of regular use. (A couple of humbly packaged and reasonably priced preparations available in drugstores and supermarkets have 8 percent AHA—considerably more than many of the fancier department store brands.) Pseudoscientific claims trumpeted in cosmetic ads or presented by models in lab coats at cosmetics counters only mislead the public and waste their money. Foundations and moisturizers that contain sunscreens actually contribute more to maintaining a youthful appearance than the low levels of AHAs in these products.

The stronger an acid, the deeper into the skin it can penetrate. In general, the fruit acids act only in the upper layers of the epidermis to dissolve the matrix that holds together individual cells in the innermost layer of the stratum corneum. This is the layer of dead skin cells that is normally shed about once a month. When this intercellular "glue" is dissolved, the cells have no attachment to one another and so can be shed more easily. Essentially, this process picks up the tempo of normal skin cell turnover that begins to slow with age and sun exposure. The AHAs also bond water in the skin and increase the amount of hyaluronic acid in the dermis, which helps keep the skin moisturized.

AHAs can improve the overall appearance of facial skin by speeding up the turnover of epidermal cells, which makes the skin look smoother and fresher. What they *can't* do is fix wrinkles and sun damage down in the dermis, where the majority of such stigmata lie. There is some evidence that chemical signals pass between the dermis and epidermis. If this is so, then it is also possible improvements in the superficial layer are communicated to the dermis, but whether this dialogue can effect visible improvements in damaged dermis is unclear.

The types of peels dermatologists use most often are stronger solutions of glycolic acid, trichloracetic acid (TCA), or phenol. Repeated 50 to 70 percent glycolic acid peels are adequate to improve the blotchiness and other pigment changes that come with mild to moderate sun damage. Most patients feel comfortable starting with a 30 to 40 percent glycolic acid wash, which is stronger than they could have at a salon yet permits them to return to work after their peel with nothing more obvious than a slightly red face.

Trichloracetic acid goes deeper and, depending upon the strength of the solution, can penetrate all the layers of the epidermis and into the mid-dermis. A 20 percent solution of TCA gives a superficial peel with only a small amount of the redness or peeling that some patients find unacceptable. A stronger solution can go much deeper. We rarely use more than 40 percent TCA for cosmetic purposes. TCA of this strength is capable of penetrating to the dermis and causing new collagen to form, which helps plump up wrinkles. (We might, however, use 100 percent TCA to treat an actinic keratosis that needs to be removed to avoid the risk of its becoming a squamous cell cancer.) TCA acts by changing the acidity of the skin cells, which, in turn, destroys their cell membranes and causes the cells to die and flake off, revealing the smoother, fresh skin beneath. There are several ways we can pretreat the skin to enhance the penetration of TCA without actually increasing the strength of the acid itself. This pretreatment removes some of the epidermis so the acid that follows will penetrate deeper and more evenly.

Phenol, which is even stronger, is essentially a toxin that attacks the cellular membranes, destroying the entire epidermis and upper dermis. It is literally a controlled chemical burn. In severe long-term sun damage, the normal architecture of the dermis is destroyed and replaced by a chaotic mass of damaged collagen and elastic fibers. Blood flow is less efficient through this tangled skein of elastic tissue, so the skin becomes sallow and loses its vibrancy. Phenol is capable of stimulating the formation of new blood vessels and new bands of dermis with a more normal structure. Elasticity, color, and texture are all improved. Because it penetrates deep, the effects of phenol peels tend to last for years.

Phenol is most useful in extremely fair-skinned people who have had sun damage, because it leaves the skin snow-white. People with medium complexions look unnaturally pasty after a phenolic acid peel and do better with another method. Loretta and I don't use phenol as commonly as we do the other peeling agents because of its toxicity to the system.

Dermabrasion is another method we can use to retexture facial skin. This technique removes the epidermis and a controlled amount of dermis. The patient is given a local anesthetic to block the sensory nerves in the facial area. Then a liquid refrigerant, like Freon, is applied to temporarily freeze the skin, so that the physician has an extremely firm surface on which to work. This degree of rigidity is essential for control. (Consider the difference between planing a wooden board or a block of gelatin.) High-speed rotating wire brushes or diamond fraise selectively plane down high areas formed by some types of scars and wrinkles. The skin is actually sanded down until it appears abraded, like a skinned knee. Dermabrasion requires great skill, since the fraise rotates at 32000 rpm and, in unskilled hands, can plane the skin too much in a short time. A week or ten days' healing is necessary following dermabrasion, during which the skin must be bandaged and kept moist and free from infection. After it has healed, a full-face dermabrasion results in a remarkably smoother, rejuvenated complexion. However, as with any of the skin resurfacing techniques, if only a small area is treated, it will be lighter than the surrounding skin. How noticeable this is depends on the patient's complexion.

"Dermabrasion sounds too scary for me to start with. I'd like to try something fairly subtle at first," Anne said after I had outlined these options. "I think I'd be more comfortable with a peel."

"There are two approaches to peels. You can have either repeated light peels, which produce a more gradual and subtle change, or you can have a moderate peel, which will produce results that are more immediately noticeable."

"I'd just as soon not do something that everyone at work will notice."

"Then I would suggest starting with a 20 percent TCA peel."

"How much is it going to hurt?"

"Most of our patients say it stings for a few moments afterward, but it's nothing unbearable. Your skin will flake and peel. You'll have a certain amount of redness for five days or a week, and then you'll have a fresh, new epidermis."

"Can anything go wrong?"

"Occasionally, people can develop areas of too much or too little pigmentation or an obvious line of demarcation between the peeled and unpeeled skin or continuing redness and irritation. Infection is theoretically a risk, but we haven't had that problem with light peels. Occasionally one of these peels will reactivate herpes, so if you've had cold sores in the past, let me know, so I can give you some medicine to prevent a flare-up."

Anne made an appointment to come back in for her peel, and she left my office looking already more enthusiastic and hopeful than when she had come in.

She returned about a week later in high spirits. "I'm very excited about this," she said. "I always grew up believing that once middle age arrived, you looked it and you had no choice. Now I feel like I may get some of those horrible lost years back again."

The nurse washed Anne's face with a special skin cleanser. Then I degreased it several times with alcohol and acetone, because any patches of oil left on her face could cause the acid to be absorbed in an irregular pattern, which could lead to pigmentary abnormalities and a poor result. After Anne's face was prepped, I applied the acid solution with Q-tips, starting at her forehead, making sure to extend it into her hairline and eyebrows and just below her jawbone, to minimize lines of demarcation. Then I applied another coat in the same sequence.

"Tell me when you can feel it stinging," I told her. I handed her a Japanese paper fan to help relieve the stinging as we went along.

"I really don't feel much yet," she said after I had applied the first layer. "My skin has always been pretty tough."

Loretta and I have both noticed that many of our patients become extra stoical when they are having a peel, fanning furiously at their faces while denying feeling any pain when it is clear they are, because they want the maximum benefit from each peel.

"Anne, I don't want to leave it on to the point the stinging becomes severe. So just tell me when you've had enough, and I'll neutralize the acid."

In a few minutes, a fine white frost appeared, indicating that the TCA had destroyed the epidermis.

"Okay, I think I've just about had it. I suddenly feel like my face is on fire," Anne said.

I neutralized the acid with a solution of sodium bicarbonate and told her to keep fanning her face for a few minutes.

"That's it?" she asked. "I thought you'd have to leave it on for twenty minutes, the way they did at my facial place."

"That's it," I said. "Over the next twenty-four to thirty-six hours your skin will feel tight and look shiny. Then it will begin to crack open and peel, rather like the peeling people have with a sunburn. You'll look older before you look younger. You'll then begin to see smoother, new skin beneath. You must keep it completely protected from the sun—the whole nine yards: SPF 30, hat, and try to stay out of the sun altogether in the middle of the day. I'd like to see you back in a week."

"While I'm here, I wanted to ask you what you could do about this nasty-looking line between my eyebrows. It makes me look so stern. I'd really like to get rid of it, and I think it's next on my wish list."

"Collagen injections are what we usually use to fill fine or deep expression lines and wrinkles."

"And what do they entail?"

"If you're interested in collagen treatments, we do two sensitivity tests four weeks apart to determine whether you're allergic to either the collagen or the local anesthetic that comes with it. If you *are* allergic, which is fairly rare, there are some new alternatives we could discuss."

Collagen injections have been used in cosmetic surgery for the past fifteen years to supplement native collagen in areas where it has been weakened by sun damage or repetitive facial movements or destroyed by injury. Collagen can also be injected into the lips to create fullness.

The collagen used in cosmetic surgery is obtained from cow skin. The collagen is purified and then the ends of the molecule, which are different in cows and humans, are cut off with an enzyme. The finished product is similar to human collagen. When injected into depressions that form at sites of collagen loss, the bovine collagen aligns itself near the patient's own collagen fibers, plumping up depressions and raising them to the level of the surrounding skin. There are two formulations of bovine collagen— Zyderm, for use in smoothing fine lines and shallow scars, and Zyplast, for filling deeper lines, wrinkles, and other defects, like severe acne scars.

When Anne Barker came for her first appointment in 1983, there were no safe alternatives to collagen. Nowadays, patients who are allergic to bovine collagen or who can't be given it, because they have an autoimmune disease like lupus or rheumatoid arthritis or are taking immunosuppressive drugs like steroids, can sometimes be treated instead with a substance called Fibrel (or they can be treated with their own autologous collagen).

Fibrel was developed for use in cosmetic surgery from a material that was used to stop bleeding during surgical procedures. It is made of gelatin and aminocaproic acid, part of the body's blood-clotting mechanism. Prior to injection, these two ingredients are mixed with the patient's own blood, which provides a clotting factor. When this mixture is injected into the dermis, the body goes to work as if it were repairing a wound. First, a clot is formed at the injection site. Then fibroblasts, the cells responsible for collagen formation, appear and begin to deposit new collagen in the area. Fibrel, which is derived from pig protein, can often be used in people who are allergic to bovine-derived collagen. It can be used for the same types of repairs as collagen and, like collagen, it must be touched up at regular intervals.

Patients whose repetitive frowning is in the process of carving deep crevasses in their foreheads may elect to have their "frown muscles" paralyzed. This is done by injecting a small amount of *botulinum toxin* into the nerve that controls these muscles. Botulinum toxin, or Botox, is prepared from one of the toxins secreted by the *Clostridium* bacterium, which causes botulism. While many patients are initially rather alarmed when I describe this technique to them, I explain that it has been used in medicine for many years to help people with various facial tics as well as wry neck, a condition in which the muscles in the neck are in a perpetual painful spasm.

"But then why don't these injections give me botulism? Isn't it kind of risky?" patients invariably want to know. The difference, I tell them, is that the toxin is injected only into one nerve, whence it does not migrate. Moreover, the amount injected is minuscule and incapable of increasing, in contrast to an active case of botulism, where the bacteria are continually reproducing and pumping out more active toxin, which eventually paralyzes all the muscles in its human hosts, often killing them.

When Anne returned a week later to have her skin checked, she was delighted with the result of her first light peel.

"That's amazing stuff!" she said. "To be honest, I wasn't expecting it to do all that much more than they had done at the salon, but this is great. When I was driving home my face felt familiar, and I couldn't identify the feeling. Then I realized it felt like it would after putting on one of those peel-off masks for oily skin that were so much fun to pick off when I was a teenager. My face felt encased in this shiny film, which I kept expecting to crack open the way those masks did. Then I had a few days when the film still hadn't started to peel off yet, but it was getting all cracked and dry. I looked in the mirror on the morning of day three, and I felt like I was getting a preview of my face in fifteen years. One of my friends took a picture of me. But then it started to flake off, and I could see that I really had lost some little lines, and my skin tone looked so much healthier and more even. And unlike the salon facials, where your skin looks good until you wake up the next day, this looks great even a week later. I'm impressed."

She paused to look again in the mirror. "You mentioned that a series of these light peels will bring the most improvement, so when can I have more? Or should I have a deeper peel?"

"A deeper peel with a stronger TCA solution would remove more of the lines on your upper lip as well as some of the brown spots that didn't improve with this peel. The other thing you need to understand is that the effects of anything but the deep resurfacing procedures are temporary. How long they last depends on how much sun damage you've accrued over the years and how well you protect your skin in the future." Usually, patients who prefer light peels come in on a continuing basis for maintenance. Although too-frequent peels may cause a breakout of acne, monthly light peels help most people maintain maximally smooth, clear skin.

"Then I want another appointment, and I think I'd like to try a deeper peel. How long do I have to wait?"

"You should wait about a month until the next one. But while you're here today, I want to talk to you about your daily skin care regimen, because there's so much you yourself can do to hold the line on aging. You seemed disappointed with all the skin care products you brought in at your first appointment, so I want to suggest a simpler, more effective—and also less expensive—program for you."

"Great. I'm so tired of going to cosmetics counters and getting talked into buying all those expensive products that don't work as well as they promise, and then going to another counter two months later and getting talked into buying a whole *other* line."

"I'm going to suggest a rinse-off cleanser followed by a 10 percent glycolic acid lotion, which you also rinse off. Then I'd like you to use a moisturizing lotion that contains glycolic acid and also a chemical called hydroquinone, which will help bleach some of your freckles and uneven pigment."

"So you believe that soap and water are the best way to clean my face? I was told a long time ago that it was better not to use soap and water, because they'd dry my skin out."

Whenever patients bring up this question, I am reminded of a patient of Loretta's, an exceptionally pretty Frenchwoman in her thirties, whose complaint was that she had suddenly developed a number of inflamed acnelike lesions on either side of her nose. It turned out that this woman's mother had told her never to use soap and water on her face. And she never had. Indeed, except for the reddened, bumpy areas, she had a classic milky-white, unlined complexion, due to her mother's accompanying injunction never to go out into the sun without a hat and long sleeves. Naturally, after having taken such scrupulous care of her skin for so many years, she was horrified at the uncontrollable outbreak sullying her complexion. Loretta cleverly had diagnosed *demodicidosis,* a disorder that arises when the sebaceous follicles are invaded by microscopic mites known as *Demodex folliculorum.* While this disease is not commonly diagnosed, it sometimes crops up in patients with an inflammatory condition of the facial skin known as *rosacea.* Loretta's patient did not have rosacea. The mites had colonized her follicles, because they enjoyed the nourishment of the rich cleansing creams she used instead of soap and water. She was utterly horrified to find out she was harboring these unattractive guests. Their presence was all it took to convince her to change her lifelong regimen to one that employed enough mild soap to make her facial environment less hospitable to the mites, by removing normal sebaceous secretions and bacteria on a regular basis.

"How you cleanse your skin depends somewhat upon your skin type and your daily activities. Since you work out at a gym and also have some oily areas around your nose and chin, I think you should use a mild detergent or soap-based cleanser at least once a day. It will help dissolve any sebum that has accumulated in your pores, and it helps keep bacteria in check, so your skin doesn't break out."

"My mother used only Pond's cold cream and tissues to clean her face, and her skin was perfect."

"Older people, whose skin tends to be dryer, and people who have smooth skin with small pores can get away without really degreasing their skin. I'm not advising you to overdry your skin, but you should give it a thorough cleansing at least once a day. If you prefer to use a cream-type cleanser, you can use it in the evening. There are a couple of commercial ones we think are particularly good."

"Since I have slightly oily skin, do I still need to use a moisturizer?"

"You do need something around the eye area. The one I'm going to suggest isn't greasy. You'll be surprised, because it feels like water going on, but you'll find it makes your skin feel moist and supple but not at all oily. If it isn't enough in the winter, you can switch to one that is a little more emollient and provides more of a barrier to the environment."

"Those cosmetics counter assistants always made such a big deal about selling me moisturizers."

"Actually, I always tell people that the ideal moisturizers for dry skin on the body, from the dermatologist's—not the cosmetician's—point of view, are Eucerin and Vaseline, but I realize they're not exactly pleasurable to use."

"I'll say!"

"I think you'd also benefit from using Retin-A at least a couple of times a week to start. You don't have extensive sun damage, but the Retin-A will help repair what you do have and prevent more wrinkles. Another thing we're finding is that it seems both to prevent skin cancer and also to keep precancerous spots from progressing to cancers."

"I've been reading about Retin-A, and I was going to ask you if I could try it. It sounds like a miracle."

"I find that many of my patients will benefit from it, but I want to make sure you understand that if you start using it, you really have to use a serious sunblock—which is to say, at least SPF 30—and a hat whenever possible. Retin-A thins the outer layers of the skin and makes you a little more sensitive to the sun. When you're putting on the sunscreen, apply it twenty minutes before you go out in the sun, so it has a chance to sink into your skin, and don't forget the backs of your hands and your neck. Even if you stop using Retin-A, remember your peels are exposing new skin, which is much more susceptible to burning and sun damage. The other thing to remember is that after peels or dermabrasion, sun exposure can cause you to develop uneven pigmentation, so you really can't be lax about your sunblock."

"That's the hard part for me. I am so delighted to have my face look less lined, but I do like getting a little color in the summer."

"Ideally, I wish my patients would just try to change their concept of what's attractive, but I realize that's easy for me to say and far less easy for people to do. The myth of a tanned, healthy glow is strongly inculcated in our minds, and it dies hard. But you can use the self-tanning products they have now."

"Oh ick!" she cried. "You mean that awful stuff they had in the sixties? That stuff that dyed you bright orange?"

"The products have gotten a lot better since then. You should try a couple of different ones and see which gives you the most natural color. Quite a few are on the market now, and people seem to have strong opinions about the different brands."

"But are these things safe?"

"Absolutely." Even though I prefer my patients to change their ideas about what constitutes a healthy-looking complexion, I'm happy to recommend self-tanners with the proviso that they use a sunblock at the same time.

Self-tanning agents work by staining the epidermis brown. While the pigmentary changes that occur following sun exposure do provide some sun protection—after the initial damage is done—the "tan" induced by self-tanners is purely a chemical reaction at the surface of the skin, which doesn't stimulate production of the protective pigment, melanin, and therefore provides no sun protection.

Anne Barker was so pleased with the results of her first two peels that she began to come in for peels every other month. Over the course of eight or nine months, her skin texture improved markedly. The fact that she hadn't sustained a great deal of sun damage made her face an excellent palette on which to work. And each time she came into the office, she looked happier and more confident. There was a glow to her face for which I could not claim credit. She began to wear eye makeup and, although she had worn the same pair of baggy corduroy trousers to her first three appointments, she began to arrive in really flattering clothes. This is a phenomenon we see repeatedly in patients who have had cosmetic procedures. As they begin to like what they see in their mirrors, they are encouraged to care for their skin better and to do all they can to enhance their appearance.

One day, after she had been coming to me for about a year, Anne showed up looking like the proverbial cat who swallowed the canary. Before I could even comment on her extra-high spirits and the Mona Lisa smile she couldn't wipe off her face, Susan, my nurse, spoke up: "Anne, you didn't come in your station wagon today!"

"What's she driving today?" I asked as I swabbed Anne's face with acid. "A red Porsche Targa?"

"Better still! *A*, she's not even driving. Some good-looking guy is. And, *B*, he's driving a big silver Rolls Royce!"

"And it sure is fun!" Anne giggled, relaxing her face so I could apply the TCA.

After that, Anne arrived frequently in the Rolls. Each time, the office staff would flock to the window to ogle the well-dressed gent at the wheel. One day, Anne called to reschedule her next appointment.

"Mr. Rolls Royce has invited me to go to Bermuda next week," she explained to the receptionist. "Tell Dr. Balin not to worry. I've got SPF 30 sunblock and a big hat. I even found some pretty gloves I can wear in the sun."

When Anne returned, I was delighted to see she had been true to her word. Her color was exactly the same as the day she had boarded the airplane to go south. This isn't always the case with my patients. All too often, even the ones who know better are unable to resist reverting to their former beach behavior and undoing much of our progress. Moreover, the damage is often more severe, because they are bombarding fresh new epidermis and newly reconstituted dermis with extra-high-intensity ultraviolet light reflecting off sand and water. I tell patients that the damage they're doing to their skin under those circumstances is akin to leaving a three-month-old baby on the beach at high noon.

The only change I noticed in Anne's skin was a splash-shaped dark patch on her forearm.

"Isn't this the weirdest thing?" she asked, pointing it out. "I was sitting in the sun *in* my sunblock, in my hat, but I was wearing a short-sleeved tennis dress. We were having margaritas, and when I went to squeeze a lime into mine, some of the juice sprayed onto my arm, and then this mark developed a few days later."

What Anne had experienced was a not uncommon photosensitivity reaction, called *berlocque dermatitis,* caused by the interaction between sunlight and a class of compounds known as psoralens. While psoralens are used therapeutically to sensitize the skin to the effects of ultraviolet light in psoriasis and vitiligo, among other conditions, such exposures are controlled by the physician. Although Anne's reaction was caused by the combination of sun and lime juice, the psoralens in perfume or aftershave containing oil of bergamot may also react with sunlight. Oil of bergamot, derived from the peel of bitter oranges, is a common component of many fragrances as well as an ingredient in Earl Grey tea. Individuals vary in their susceptibility to berlocque dermatitis, but it's better not to wear perfume or aftershave on exposed areas of the skin when venturing out in the sun.

After explaining this to Anne, I said, "This mark will fade in a couple of months, but if it bothers you, there's some good camouflage makeup available."

"Oh no, it really doesn't bother me. I was just curious what had caused it. I'm glad I didn't get it around my mouth, like a mustache! Speaking of which, I think now's the time for some collagen. I'd really like to get rid of these lines above my lips. The peels have improved them a lot, but I've got to tell you, I had the shock of my life on the plane, when I looked at myself in the unflattering light of one of those awful bathrooms. I saw lines I had never seen before, and I saw my lipstick is getting wicked up into those rays around my mouth. For me, that's the limit. That's real grandmother stuff!"

That day, after I had performed Anne's regular peel, I injected a small amount of collagen into her forearm. "I want you to come in next week, so I can take a look at this patch," I said, "and I want you yourself to keep an eye out for any redness or swelling or itching. I'll do another sensitivity test in a month, just to be certain you're not sensitive to collagen. If you are, we can try the Fibrel, or we can do an autologous collagen transfer."

The patch test showed that Anne was not sensitive to either lidocaine or bovine collagen, so she began the next phase of her desired transformation. Anne Barker was a good candidate for collagen augmentation, because she had sustained so little sun damage that her skin had retained its youthful, healthy elasticity.

"One of my friends who has had these collagen injections said the ones into the upper lip hurt the most," Anne said nervously, eyeing the hypodermic.

"They do hurt a little," I agreed, "but what I'm injecting contains some local anesthetic along with the collagen, and most people find they actually don't end up hurting as much as they're afraid they will."

I carefully injected the contents of the syringe, which is one-third collagen and two-thirds salt water, through overlapping punctures into the most superficial layer of Anne's dermis. Because only about a third of the injected filler remains in place, it is necessary to add extra and overcorrect the area. After I had finished, Anne asked for a mirror.

"Uh-oh!" she cried, running her finger over her lip. "I'm not sure I like this. I knew my lip would be swollen, but it looks enormous!"

"Don't worry, the swelling will disappear in a day or two. Remember I told you I would have to inject a little extra because of the salt water? That's what you're feeling. Soon the extra fluid will disappear, and your lip will look the way you expect it to."

"How long will this last?"

"Most people find they want touch-ups with smaller amounts of collagen anywhere from four to six months after their initial treatment, but it depends somewhat on your expectations. Areas that aren't subjected to a lot of movement can last for up to two years. If that happens, of course, the correction may last a good deal longer."

Because injected collagen is virtually identical to that which is contained in human dermis, it, too, is subject to the same mechanical forces that can cause native collagen to wear down, including smiling, smoking, and other repetitive facial muscle movements.

Anne called the office a few days later to say that the swelling and redness were gone and her upper lip had lost the scored look that she found so ugly.

"I remember seeing lines like that on some of my mother's friends and thinking their upper lips looked like cube steaks, but I didn't realize until recently how bad mine were, too. What I like best of all is that my lipstick now stays where it's supposed to, instead of a quarter of an inch away."

Anne had saved up so many weeks of vacation time at her job during the years after her withdrawal from life that she decided to take a month off to go to Seattle to visit her brother and his family, something she hadn't done since her son's death.

"You sure can't beat waking up in the morning and liking what you see in the mirror," she told me when she came in for her last pre-vacation peel. "I remember my first appointment, where you warned me not to expect a few cosmetic improvements to change my life, but you were being too conservative. They really have changed my life. I call it my renaissance."

The transformation Jay McClane sought that summer while Anne was away was merely to be made recognizable again. When I first met Mr. McClane, I was struck by his resemblance to W. C. Fields. The major part of this visual similarity was contributed by his red, bulbous nose. Touchingly, he had brought with him to our first meeting a photograph taken some fifty years before, in the army. That old sepia-toned black-and-white portrait showed a jaunty young man in khaki with the rakish confidence of a young Jimmy Cagney. He was dark-haired and handsome, with that mildly flattened pugilist's nose so many women seem to find irresistible. What a contrast to the grandfather sitting in my office half a century further on in his life.

"Doc, I hope you can help me, because I'm beginning to feel like I don't even want to go outside anymore. I'm not a vain person, but all I can think of to do now is hide out where no one can see me."

It was easy to see why. From the front, Jay's nose appeared

merely large, red, and lumpy. But, from the side, it was protuberant and pendulous. Studded throughout its pachydermatous folds were enlarged follicles encrusted with white cellular debris and sebum. The growth itself extended in a cauliflower-like mass nearly an inch from the tip of his actual nose. I could see immediately that Jay was suffering from a condition called *rhinophyma.*

Although rhinophyma is primarily a disease of middle-aged and elderly men, it usually arises from a disease called rosacea, which can afflict both sexes. Rosacea generally first strikes people in their thirties and forties. It is more common in fair-complected people and those who blush easily or frequently. Rosacea, also referred to as acne rosacea, appears like a perpetual deep blush, although red lesions resembling those of acne may appear on the cheeks and chin. Unlike acne vulgaris, however, rosacea is not due to overactive sebaceous glands, and people with rosacea do not have blackheads. The flush of rosacea is due to telangiectasias, or enlarged blood vessels, in the upper dermis. These knots of dilated veins are often mistakenly referred to as broken blood vessels or spider veins. People with rosacea may suffer only the occasional flare-up of these dilated vessels, whereas those who have developed telangiectasias due to solar damage have them permanently unless they are treated.

Rosacea is a fairly mysterious disorder, and it can be extremely difficult to control, a source of frustration for patients, particularly young women. It's especially stigmatizing because untrained eyes frequently mistake its flush for that of alcoholism. While it is true that alcohol, temperature extremes, and spicy foods may aggravate rosacea by dilating the dermal blood vessels, the redness is not caused by chronic drinking. Plenty of people with rosacea never touch a drop. (It is true, however, that liver disease may cause telangiectasias to appear on the face.) Many culprits have been suspected, but no one yet knows what causes rosacea. It is likely that there is no single trigger. Although rosacea is not a bacterial disease, it, like acne, frequently responds to oral tetracyclines, which in this case have an anti-inflammatory effect. A topical preparation of the antimicrobial drug metronidazole is also commonly and sometimes successfully used to treat rosacea. The main thing is that rosacea warrants treatment to prevent it from progressing to its most disfiguring form.

"I always looked kinda red in the face, but I figured it was because I'm Irish and I like to drink," Jay confided. "I don't drink much more than beer anymore, but I used to like to tie one on pretty good after work when I was a doorman in New York City. Most of us who worked in the neighborhood liked to stop in at a place around the corner for a couple of shots and beers before we headed home. I thought maybe when I stopped drinking my face would stop being so red, but it never did. Then, after a while, this thing started growing on my nose. It started out as a red lump about ten years ago, and it's been getting bigger ever since. Like I said, I'm not a vain person, but I like to be around people, and I want them to like me, not be disgusted."

I nodded in sympathy. His expression was so pained, I was glad I was going to be able to give him the good news that I could restore his nose to near normal without much difficulty.

"I think what finally made me come in was the other day I overheard my little grandson—he's six years old—tell his mother he didn't want to sit on my lap, because my nose looked like popcorn and he didn't want me to touch him. That kinda hurt, because that little fellow means the world to me. I want us to be pals." Tears came to his eyes, and he swiped at them in embarrassment.

After examining Mr. McClane, I explained to him that although the rosacea on his cheeks might continue to flare up periodically even with treatment, I could return his nose to normal. The whole surgical procedure could be done in the office under local anesthesia.

"You're kidding!" he cried in relief. "I was kind of worried I'd be stuck with this for good. I'm glad I came."

When Mr. McClane returned for his surgery, I removed the excess tissue under local anesthesia, and he went home with a nearly normal nose beneath his dressings.

"Doc, you've made me feel like a member of the human race again," he said when he came in for me to check his progress. "You have no idea what it was like always feeling so ashamed to be seen."

I still see Jay McClane from time to time for other problems. Like many blue-eyed people of Celtic ancestry who have spent time in the sun, Mr. McClane developed some skin cancers and precancerous actinic keratoses. In going through his chart, I often look at the "before" and "after" pictures from his first visits. While the first photographs show a man facing the camera with hesitancy and shame, those taken two weeks later depict a different man—one facing the camera forthrightly, with just the shadow of a smile playing across his face.

When Anne Barker returned in the fall for a peel, I again rechecked her entire body for any suspicious-looking moles. One on her back, which I had earlier noted in her chart, had grown a little, and I decided it would be best to remove and biopsy it.

"You've been very good about using sunblock, I see, but since you wear your hair short, don't forget to protect the back of your neck," I warned. Sometimes I see farmers and other outdoor workers whose major sun damage is on the back of their necks, where the sun has beaten down for years without so much as the bill of a cap to shield it—hence the disparaging term "redneck."

When Anne's biopsy report was returned to me, it said her mole was what is known as a *dysplastic nevus*. Although this is not a cancerous lesion, it is a warning sign. People who have dysplastic nevi have a tenfold increased risk of developing a melanoma. I explained this to Anne and described for her the warning signs to watch out for. Dysplastic nevi, like melanomas, are unevenly colored, often with a lighter edge around a darker center, and are generally larger than other moles.

"It's a good idea, Anne, for you to check your moles frequently yourself. I have been checking them every six months, and I will continue to, but I always suggest to patients that they also keep an eye out for changes."

"That brings me to another question, Dr. Balin. I've decided to move to Seattle for a while. I'm going to lease out my house here for a year and give it a try. I found I liked being out there with my nieces and nephews, and I think it might be the final step I need to really put the past behind me. Is there a dermatologist you could refer me to out there who could at least continue with the TCA peels and keep an eye on the rest of my skin?"

"Of course. Let me make some phone calls, and I'll get some names for you. By the way, congratulations on your decision. I wish you all the best. We'll miss you."

"You know, Dr. Balin, I really have you to thank for my renaissance. Oh, I know I've done a lot of the work myself, but it never would have happened so quickly if you hadn't done such a great job of giving me back some of those lost years."

"Thank you for the compliment, but don't forget that you came to me. You were ready."

"Oh well, it's a chicken-and-egg thing, I suppose. But this did change my life. It got me over my depression, and I'm looking forward to a fresh start at age forty-seven. Don't ever let anyone tell you that cosmetic changes are only skin deep."

Anne returned to see me about a year later.

"I'm back to sell my house," she explained. "I've met a wonderful guy, and we're going to be married on New Year's Eve. Before I go, I'd like you to fix a couple of last things. One is my thighs. I really want liposuction. Another is my hands, and the last is that furrow between my eyebrows. My doctor in Seattle has been giving me collagen injections, and I get great results for a while, but I've already had it done twice, and it's expensive. Isn't there anything else we could try that would last better?"

"There is a new technique using a material called Gore-Tex instead of collagen."

"I think I have a Gore-Tex ski parka," she replied looking puzzled. "It's great stuff, but do I really want it in my face?"

Gore-Tex is a manmade material first introduced to medicine nearly twenty-five years ago, when it was used to patch blood vessels in vascular surgery. It was an ideal material for this purpose, since it is physiologically inert, meaning that it doesn't cause allergic or toxic reactions and can't be absorbed and degraded by the body. It is elastic enough to expand and contract with the pulsatile flow of blood coursing through the circulatory system. In dermatology, it has the benefit of being smooth and soft, and it can be placed below the dermis, in the fatty layer. This allows it to plump up some of the deepest facial expression lines, like the "marionette lines" that extend from the mouth to the chin, and the nasolabial folds, from the nose to the lips. It's an outpatient procedure, in which a small incision is made at each end of the wrinkle one wants to fill in. A needlelike instrument is used to pull a small strip of Gore-Tex through the incision and position it beneath the wrinkle. The result is instantaneous and causes little discomfort to the patient.

"That sounds interesting. At least you could do it before I left and not have to touch it up."

"Theoretically it is a good idea, but it's not one I would recommend for you at the moment. Your lines aren't deep enough yet. You'd really be better off sticking with collagen."

So far, I believe that injected bovine collagen or autocollagen, which is collagen harvested from a patient's own skin, is the safest, simplest, most effective way of filling in facial lines, even if it is less than permanent. Loretta and I are experimenting with some line-filling techniques of our own that we hope will overcome the problems of foreign-body reactions and the need for repeated touch-ups.

"All right, you've convinced me to stay with the collagen for the moment," she said. "Now, what about my hands?"

"What is it about them you would like to change?" I asked.

She stretched them out in front of her. "In my business, so many people see my hands, and they look so bony and veiny and old. They remind me of my grandmother's hands. Mine don't have as many liver spots as hers did, but I'd like to get rid of the ones I do have."

"The best way of rejuvenating your hands would be to do an autologous fat transfer, which means we remove some of your own fat with a syringe and inject it into the fatty layer below the dermis of your hands."

"Can't you use some of the fat you take out of my thighs? I'm sure there'll be plenty of it!"

"I'd use a suction device to remove the fat from your hips and thighs. That fat can't be reused, because it gets damaged and contaminated in the suction machine. But what I can do is remove some of the fat from your thighs with a syringe, before I use the machine, and reinject it in your hands. Just as with the collagen injections into your lips, I'd have to overcorrect your hands and put in quite a lot of extra fat, because eventually 80 percent of it will die and be reabsorbed, and only 20 percent will take and live."

"And then after you did that, how would you get rid of the liver spots?"

"We could freeze them off with liquid nitrogen or carbon dioxide snow. We could also remove them with a Q-switch neodymium YAG laser, which would give the best cosmetic result. This laser specifically targets and destroys the brown melanin in the skin."

We are currently using the Ultrapulse CO_2 laser on patients who have wrinkles and/or extensive sun damage and want to rejuvenate their skin in a noticeable way. We like it because it does the same excellent resurfacing job that dermabrasion does, except that it is much easier for us to control than high-speed rotating brushes, and it's less painful for patients. It's not an inexpensive technology, so many of our patients continue to have peels instead, but its results are spectacular. With it, we can remove lines and brown spots of various sorts and really subtract twenty years from many faces. And while it gives a fresh new canvas of smooth, youthful skin, it doesn't obliterate all the expression lines, which many patients feel are appropriate and desirable. Loretta and I both agree that these lines are important communicators of the personality and spirit within each person. With the laser, we can give the patients the best of both worlds: perfect skin and a face that retains its unique character.

"Since I am on a bit of a budget now that I have a husband to consider too, I want to go home and think about what I really want done."

She called a few days later. "I've managed to convince myself that my hands are actually sensitive and artistic-looking. If I can just get the brown spots off them, then I think I can do without the fat transfer. What I really want to concentrate on is getting rid of those hideous saddlebags on my thighs."

Humans are born with a genetically determined number of potential fat cells, which increase in number through infancy and then cease production. Weight gain after this time is due to an enlargement of the fat cells rather than an increase in their number. Fat cells can enlarge to many times their normal size, permitting enormous weight gain. Diet and exercise can reduce the size of fat cells, but their number can be reduced only by actually removing them. Once removed, they do not grow back. While dieting and exercise may suffice to produce a desirable figure in many people, others find that their fat is distributed unevenly, so that a woman with a slim rib cage and long, thin extremities may be tortured by having the hips, thighs, and buttocks of a Rubens courtesan. Or a man with a generally slender build may develop fatty breasts or a stubborn paunch. These disproportionate fat deposits can occur because of differences in the metabolism of fat cells in different locations. Our figure is partly inherited. The body that begins to take shape in middle age may be doing so nearly independently of diet and exercise as we grow into an inherited template.

Liposuction can sculpt the body in such a way as to restore or create harmonious proportions. Disproportionately fatty areas can be whittled down to a dimension more consonant with the rest of the body. Hips, thighs, jowls, chests, knees, buttocks, all may be reshaped through liposuction.

Although liposuction has been available for some time, it used to be considered a fairly radical way of permanently removing fat from the body. It was quite a bloody procedure and not without risk. Nowadays, thanks to modifications in the technique developed by Dr. Jeff Klein, a dermatologist, liposuction can be performed painlessly and virtually bloodlessly in a doctor's office.

As I carefully marked on Anne's skin the areas where I planned to insert the cannula, she shivered nervously. "Now I'm getting kind of scared. One part of me would be willing to submit to any torture just to be able to have normal thighs that don't look like I'm wearing riding jodhpurs all the time, and part of me is ready to faint dead away just thinking about what you're going to be doing."

"Don't worry, Anne," my nurse, Eileen, piped in. "Dr. Balin removed 800 cc's of fat from my inner thighs, and I barely knew when he was doing it. Really. All I felt was a little tugging, and I can promise you I have no pain tolerance at all. It's great. In two days you won't believe your eyes."

After I had finished removing the fat from the various areas I had marked on Anne's outer thighs and buttocks, which took about two hours, I put one stitch across each of the minute incisions I had made for inserting the cannula and dressed them. I then applied a pressure bandage to the entire area I had worked on. For the first few days after liposuction, the patient wears a specially designed girdle or some other type of elastic dressing that will put pressure on the treated area. This is done to reduce swelling and allow the remaining fat to reshape itself. After two weeks, most patients, if they have developed bruising, will have little left, and they will be able to see the expected results. In many patients, the treated area continues to shrink up to six months after the surgery. This probably happens because fat cells adjacent to those suctioned away are themselves damaged and eventually eliminated by the body.

The lipoinjection technique Anne considered for rejuvenating her hands can also be used for body sculpting by putting back or shoring up what gravity has made fall. In the past, facelifts were all that was available to revitalize a face. The procedure involved cutting away excess skin and then redraping what was left. Invariably, it resulted in an instantly identifiable, drawn, masklike look. But faces can age in different ways. For those whose facial aging is due more to loss of the subcutaneous fat pad and a shrinking skeleton, replacing lost fat rather than cutting skin and redraping the facial skin is a far more subtle and natural way of rebuilding youthful contours using a patient's own (autologous) fat tissue. Instead of an operation in a hospital under general anesthesia, liposculpture can safely be done in the office. Since 80 percent of the injected fat will be reabsorbed, we overcorrect slightly. Usually two or more treatments are needed to accumulate enough fat that "takes" and remains in place.

At her last visit before she was to leave for her new life in Seattle, Anne shook my hand good-bye. "You know, Arthur," she said. "At first I couldn't decide whether I should see a psychotherapist or a dermatologist, and I came to see you because I didn't want to sit and endlessly rehash the past. I wanted to embrace the future and get on with my life. I didn't care what some of my friends started to say about my being addicted to cosmetic surgery. What, I asked them, is so wrong with looking in the mirror and looking like you've got as much life left as you feel you have? Now I look in the mirror, and the inside and the outside match!"

She then went on to describe to me a study she had read about by psychologist Dr. Ellen Langer and her colleagues at Harvard, in which two groups of healthy elderly men were sent on a retreat. One group merely went on a pleasant country vacation where they could unwind for a week. The others did the same, but they were also put into a virtual time warp. They weren't allowed to bring with them anything—books, newspapers, photographs—dated after 1959. The newspapers they read were those of forty years in the past; the current events they discussed at dinner were of that era. They wore the types of clothes they had in their twenties; they listened to the old songs. Their conversations described young wives and children, careers still in full swing. Their environment was totally manipulated to mimic the world that had existed when they were in their fifties. They lived this way for a week. During the retreat, each man underwent a series of tests of strength, posture, endurance, cognition, and memory as well as sight, taste, and hearing, with the purpose of establishing an estimated biologic age.

"What was really amazing, I thought, was that in comparison to the other group, who just went on a restful retreat and talked about the past as though it were past, the time-warp group really changed," Anne said. "Testers who looked at their 'before' and 'after' pictures said the men in the time-warp group looked an average of three years younger. Their posture straightened, their vision improved, their grip strength improved; even their intelligence test scores were slightly better.

"When I read that, Arthur, I suddenly realized that I was doing the right thing for myself. If the face you look at every morning in the mirror looks like that of your mother or grandmother or some other older lady, you start to feel older inside than you need to, and then you begin first to act that way, and then you actually become that way. I remember the day I came home after having that first peel and I looked in the mirror and I suddenly felt like I had gone back in time, because I was looking at a slightly younger version of myself—an Anne who had been. As I started to lose those lines and my skin started to glow again, I began to look like the Anne I remembered from ten years ago, and I think that had a powerful effect on how I felt and behaved. It was as though I hadn't really lost those years after Tommy's death. When I read about that study, it made so much sense to me."

In a way, Anne was reiterating what my father had said when he wanted me to lift his neck. "Why should I look any older than I feel?" Our outsides and our insides may age at vastly different rates. The woman whose chronologic age is forty and whose biologic age is actually ten years older than that may be looking into the mirror and seeing a woman in her late fifties. Rather than truly reflecting her age—either chronologic or biologic—this image in the mirror is merely reflecting accumulated environmental damage. Eventually, she comes to feel more like the face in the mirror than the energetic young girl still inside her. I believe very much in the power of hypnosis in medicine. One of the tenets of hypnotherapy is that the body cannot distinguish between something truly experienced and something vividly imagined. Thus, to confront a rejuvenated face in the mirror every day and feel as if one has traveled back into one's own life may indeed have the power to rejuvenate the body and spirit to some degree as well. Perhaps therein lies the true gift of cosmetic surgery—the ability to make consonant the outer and inner person and perhaps slow the rate of aging. I consider that powerful medicine.

My Father's Facelift
and Other Family
Matters

―――― ⦿⦿ ――――

As the flight attendant stopped by my seat to remind me to stow my briefcase for takeoff, I realized I had been staring out at the runway for the half hour I'd been on board. I had started out by going over in my mind the key points I wanted to make in my opening remarks the next day as chair of a conference on aging, but from there my thoughts had wandered. First they touched on each of the whole roster of topics under the heading "Things I Want to Do When I Have Time" that I keep stored away in the back of my mind. At the head of the list was the tenth or so self-reminder that I wanted to bring home one of the extra cryostats I have at the office, for making paper-thin slices of leaves and bugs and other such things, which I could video through my microscope and project on television for Allison and her baby brother, Benjamin. I had spent a good deal of the previous Sunday afternoon walking around our property towed by three-year-old Allison who, to my delight, was entering the "Why?" stage so many parents find exasperating. It would be fun to set up a small home lab so I could explore the mysteries of science with my children right from the start. When I was a child, I built a research

lab in my parents' basement and played in it most of my childhood, adding to it and making it more sophisticated as I learned
more.

"All right," Loretta said warily when I told her my idea. "But I
don't want you trying to influence Allison into becoming a scientist or anything else at this stage. I want her to discover for herself
what interests her. Just because you've been a doctor since the age
of three . . ."

I smiled. I knew where Loretta had gotten *that* line. It's one of
my mother's favorites. In actual fact, I can't remember any of the
occasions when I attempted to take my father's pulse or put ointment on one of my mother's cuts. I do have a vague recollection
that at around age nine, when I had an aquarium, I became quite
interested in fish diseases. This was really a matter of expediency,
because tropical fish were expensive to replace from my allow-
ance. I found a book on fish diseases, studied it, and then apparently hired myself out around the neighborhood as a fish
physician, or so my mother says. When I got my medical degree, I
remember various of my parents' friends coming up and asking
me if I remembered the time when I came over and set up an
isolation ward for their zebra fish or cured their black mollies of
some fungus and telling me they knew then that I was destined to
become a doctor. I nod politely, but I really don't remember.

I do remember that in my freshman year in high school, after
spending a couple of years helping with autopsies at a local hospital and various hospital lab tests, like blood cell counts, I acquired
a *Merck Manual,* with which I "diagnosed" and sometimes
"treated" the various maladies my friends presented to me. My
father recently reminded me of a couple of misdiagnoses I made.
Fortunately, in both cases I must have realized I was a bit over my
head. When I called my father for a consult I found that both
patients needed to see a *real* doctor—stat.

I think the beginnings of my scientific career came with my
discovery of the Tom Swift books when I was about ten. I would
bet that if one took a poll of the male scientists and doctors of a
certain age in this country, more than a few would say their scientific imaginations had been fired by Tom Swift. I know I read each
of the books at least ten times. I still have them stored away. My

son Sam didn't share my rapture with them, but I'm hoping that if not Allison, then Ben, the baby, will find some of the same excitement in those books that I did.

I wanted to tell Loretta that I wasn't trying to influence Allison to become anything in particular, although I am not sure it's completely true. I certainly want to share with her at this magical time in her life and at this time in the history of science some of the exquisite beauty of the world around her. But to be completely honest, I'd have to say I *do* want to influence her, at least indirectly, because she already seems to have an interest. Even Loretta admits Allison already has a medical bent. A few months after her second birthday, I was watching her eat dinner in her high chair—something I arrive home too late to do on most nights. Loretta was flipping through the channels on the television to see if she could find anything appropriate for Allison to watch. At one point, she clicked onto what appeared to be open-heart surgery in progress, with a patient laid out and slit down the middle, from xiphoid process to pubic symphysis, and clearly crashing in a fountain of blood. Loretta quickly went on, but Allison immediately began to beat her spoon and shriek, "But I *want* to see the boo-boo!" with great enthusiasm. Loretta and I exchanged glances and both shook our heads.

What I really wish for my children is that they can share Loretta's and my great luck in having the kind of work that makes us want to get up in the morning and get right back to it. Although I grew up surrounded by doctors (my father, his three brothers, and his two sisters), I found my way into science as one finds one's way through an enchanted forest. Like many inquisitive small boys of a certain bent, I was fascinated by blowing things up. I remember manufacturing ink in my lab and having my little brother, who is now involved in the financial world, go to the neighbors and sell it. The more I learned about the way things worked, the more questions I had and the more experiments I thought of to give me answers. When I was about twelve, I got an unpaid job assisting the pathologist at a local hospital in performing autopsies. When I was seventeen, I used these same skills to dismantle and rebuild, with a lot of fancy extra additions, the brand new Mustang my parents had given me. I couldn't stop. I don't even remember making the decision to go to medical school. That, for me, was a

given. The decisions revolved around how many other things outside medicine I'd have time to learn about and where best to direct
my research energies.

Loretta, on the other hand, was less certain about her path.
Although she was a graduate of the Bronx High School of Science
and did pre-med at Barnard College, she was still considering
other directions—literature, psychology, perhaps philosophy.

Loretta's future was decided in a brief moment with her terminally ill father. During his long illness, Loretta and her brother
and sisters stopped in to visit their father in the hospital at some
point every day. On this particular evening, all the children were
gathered in his room at the same time. When it came time for
them to go, Mr. Pratt said good night to each child in turn. Loretta
was last. Instead of bidding her good night by name, as he had the
others, he turned to her and said, "Doctor, I have a terrible pain in
my ankle. Can you help me?" When Loretta told me that nearly a
decade later, she said she could still feel the goosebumps she had
felt sitting there with her father. She said it was as though in his
failing state he had become clairvoyant and could see her life.

Loretta's father never lived to see her go on to become the
wonderful doctor she is. I, on the other hand, have on several
occasions had the opportunity to be my own father's doctor. It is a
fairly strict convention in medicine that one doesn't treat one's
own family members. In doing so anyway, one is crossing a recognized barrier.

It began when I saw a spot on my father's forehead and told
him it ought to be biopsied. He came in for an appointment with
me in what had been for many years his own office. I shaved a
minute piece of skin and sent it off to an experienced
dermatopathology lab for diagnosis. The report that came back
said my father had skin cancer.

I had been more or less on autopilot when I noticed his suspi-
cious spot and biopsied it. But now I was faced with a dilemma.
Should I defy convention and operate on my own father, or should
I send him to someone I trusted who could also remove it by Mohs
surgery? After changing my mind several times, I decided to ask
Loretta what she thought.

To my surprise, she said, "Why not? Otherwise, he's going to
have to go into the city. What's stopping you?"

"I'm not really sure."

"It's not like you're wondering whether you should do a kidney transplant on your own father," she replied. "This is what you do every day, and you'll do your usual good job. It seems ridiculous for him to have to go all the way to New York to find another Mohs surgeon."

My parents both echoed Loretta's sentiments. I metamorphosed from son to doctor as quickly and thoroughly as I could and went to work removing and repairing his cancer. As soon as I had begun the operation, I realized I wouldn't have wanted to entrust my father to anyone else. I had seen too many people come in for the removal of cancers that had been repeatedly "removed" using techniques other than Mohs. It's an almost daily occurrence. Recently, for example, I saw an elderly gentleman who had watched the same cancer appear and be cut from his face for two decades. In the same week, a local plastic surgeon referred a man whose own son, a dermatologist, had failed to diagnose a squamous cell cancer on his thumb for so long that it had invaded down to the bone. By the time I got to its roots, I had removed most of the man's thumb, layer by layer.

To my surprise, I found something satisfying in being the doctor with the answers for the man who, besides being my father, was my first model of a doctor and all it meant. My father was a true old-fashioned family doctor, practicing at a time when first the sulfa drugs and then antibiotics were the big advances of the day. He did house calls in all weather, delivered babies at home in the middle of the night, and stood watch by many a deathbed. My mother was right there with him, running all the nonmedical aspects of his practice like a Prussian general. There was, for me, something extra satisfying, and moving as well, in being able to be the next generation, carrying on a tradition in an era of highly specialized medicine.

After that initial crossing into unsanctioned territory, it became routine for me to examine his skin for suspicious spots. One day, when we were sailing in Florida, I noticed a large scaly area on his leg that was almost certainly a cancer.

"What's that?" I asked him, pointing at it.

He looked down. "I've never noticed that before. Maybe I

knocked it against something, or maybe it's a fungus infection. What do you think? You're the dermatologist."

A fungus infection indeed! For a moment I forgot that this poor diagnostician was my own father, whose specialty was family practice and, later, weight control.

"I think I ought to biopsy it," I said to him.

I did, and it turned out to be a squamous cell cancer, like several of the others he had had. Squamous cell cancer is between basal cell cancer and melanomas in gravity. While basal cell cancer can spread locally, even to the point where it can be extremely disfiguring—eating away, for example, until a patient actually loses her nose—it doesn't metastasize. Melanomas, once they have invaded to the point where they reach the blood or lymphatic circulation, can metastasize like wildfire and are quickly fatal. Although a squamous cell cancer shares the melanoma's capability of metastasizing, it's almost always a more indolent cancer, spreading fairly slowly.

I could see that after I had removed this newest cancer my father would be left with a rather substantial crater on his calf. Normally, I'd repair something that large by taking a graft from my patient's hip or thigh or buttock, but as I explored the skin of his hip with such a possibility in mind, he spoke up.

"You know, Arthur, I'd really like to get rid of this cockscomb under my chin," he said, taking hold of the loose flesh beneath his jaw. "It's not so bad if I stretch my neck up, but look what happens if I look down. It hangs down to my clavicle. Do you think it would be possible to cut it off and use that skin for the graft on my leg?"

I thought for a moment. It was like a problem in upholstering or dressmaking: would I have enough skin in the right shape to patch his leg? Or would the pieces I'd remove to tighten his neck be too narrow?

"I'd have to think about how to do it," I replied.

"Well, I hope you can find a way to make it work," he said. "Some people might not care, or they might figure, 'Why bother at age seventy-seven?' But to me, it's like having a disease to look in the mirror and not like what I see—not even *recognize* what I see, for that matter."

"Sure, I can understand that," I said, even though I doubt I'll be as concerned about my appearance when I'm his age. My father has always tried to maintain his good looks. Way before most men, even movie stars, were having cosmetic surgery, my father was experimenting with hair transplants and blepharoplasty to tighten the loosening skin of his upper eyelid.

"You know, looking in the mirror and feeling old and ugly is like going out with your golfing buddies and finding out your game's gone way downhill. It's depressing! It won't happen to you, because you stayed out of the sun, but I didn't know to do that."

"Are you sure you want me to use that neck skin? You know, you might end up with hair growing out of your ankle."

"I'll wear socks," he said, laughing at the image of a bearded ankle.

In the end, I did solve the technical problems. I figured I would have enough skin from his neck to repair what could turn out to be a fairly large spot on his ankle. Facial skin cancers are often so located that their removal amounts to a mini-facelift, in that I remove an area of skin and then, in the course of repairing the incision, I can't help but tighten the surrounding skin to make the pieces fit again. But in this case, I was doing more. I was performing a cosmetic procedure in order to obtain a skin graft needed for the cancer repair. It was actually a rather creative solution my father had dreamt up, and one I realized I ought to offer to other patients who might be happy to have a little nipping and tucking along with a medically necessary procedure.

I scheduled my father to be my first patient early one Saturday morning. I began the removal of his cancer by marking the area with a pen. This was so that both Izzie, the technician who would prepare the slides, and I would know exactly how the tissue specimen was oriented in relationship to the surrounding area and exactly where the cancer was. This was particularly important if I didn't get all the cancer roots on the first pass and needed to go back in and remove another layer of skin. I had already done several Mohs surgeries on my father by this point, so this part of our weekend as doctor and patient felt routine, but as I numbed his leg and prepared to remove his cancer I thought ahead to the next week, when I would be performing cosmetic surgery on my father. I glanced up at the aging neck he wanted me to fix, and for a moment I felt a poignant sadness shoot through me. I looked at the festoons of loose skin and saw in my mind that same neck from the viewpoint of an eight-year-old crewing on his father's sailboat. Forty years earlier, that neck was smooth and muscular where it ascended through the open neck of a shirt as he glanced up at the sail, pushed the tiller, and brought the boat about. He was a young man then, younger than I am now, and he seemed to me omnipotent in all the arenas of his life, whether saving lives or effortlessly commanding his sailboat. I never thought about my father growing old. It had happened imperceptibly, but that strong young neck had vanished. Almost unconsciously I felt along my own jawline. Would it undergo the same metamorphosis? Was I seeing my own neck far down the line? I thought not. I have always been an assiduous sun avoider, and besides that, so much of my life takes place indoors, in labs and treatment rooms. It made me sad my father's generation hadn't known to avoid the sun. It is always a bittersweet turning point in a child's life when he realizes that his knowledge, in some areas at least, has surpassed his parents'.

I turned my attention back to that day's job: removing all of the cancer. Dad knew the drill well. After removing what I hoped was the entire cancer, I put a dressing on his leg and took the excised bit of skin down to the lab to be stained and examined. Normally, at this point, any other patient would go back to the waiting room or back home for a few hours, until it was determined whether I'd removed all the cancer's roots. If I had, the patient wouldn't need to return until the next day, when I would repair the incision. If I hadn't, he or she would return for more cutting. Sometimes the cancers were so big that people would have to return four or more times.

"You can just stay put," I told him. "Izzie's making your slides up right now. Unless, of course, you want to come down to the lab and look at them," I added. Even though he was my father, as men of medicine we were peers, and I liked that.

"I've seen enough of my own skin cancers. I'll just stay here and read my book," he replied affably. "It's kind of fun to be a patient here after all these years. You know, I always liked this corner examining room the best. It was always a little easier to work in. Of course," he said, glancing around at the various gadgets I had, "you've got so much more equipment in here than I ever did. I don't know how you can move around." I could remember his examining rooms well. They were typical of his era—an examining table, a stool, a scale, and some cabinets on the wall. Of course, he wasn't running an outpatient operating room. I had to have monitoring equipment and all the surgical tools of my trade.

It turned out to be a long day. I had to remove four layers of skin before I reached the healthy skin below the cancer's roots.

"We can go home, finally," I told him. "I got it all. Let me just tape down that dressing a little better. Mom's gone out to warm up the car for you. I'll see you next week, unless you have any problems in between. You know where to reach me."

"You mean I don't have to call your answering service, Doctor?" he joked.

Usually I can repair my Mohs surgery patients the day after the cancer is removed, but with large cancers like the one on my father's leg, which require a graft, I usually wait four or five days, until some healing has begun and a bed of new blood vessels begins to form so the graft can be easily nourished. The night before I was to do the neck lift and the graft, I sat up late with my father's neck photographs in front of me. I marked in ink where I would make the incisions. I was surprised at myself. This was an operation I knew how to do in my sleep, yet I realized I was feeling nervous. As much as I tried to tell myself that working on my father was the same as working on any other patient, it wasn't at all. Even though I had been a doctor for over twenty years, there was still an element of childhood, of bringing home my report card for his approval, in the situation.

The next morning, as the nurses prepped my father and laid out all the instruments I'd need for the different procedures I'd be performing, my father looked up at me and said, "You know Arthur, I'm really delighted this worked out. There's no one else I'd rather have doing this job."

I didn't know what to say back, but his words pleased me. I switched on the radio. "Do you have any preference as to music?"

"I'd prefer classical," said my father who, to my ears, could just about rival Segovia on the guitar. "Unless you have some educational tape you want to hear. I enjoy those too. They're a good way for me to keep up. I like to have some idea what you younger doctors are thinking."

I always defer to my patients' choice of music. Fortunately, since the patients I operate on tend to be older people, I've never had a patient request rock and roll, which might be difficult to work to. In many cases, my patients are happy to listen to audiotapes of medical meetings and other educational programs.

I began the day's work by liposuctioning the fat under my father's chin, using the new Klein-tumescent technique. This technique has revolutionized liposuction, changing it from a risky, bloody operation that could be quite harmful to one that can be performed safely and painlessly in the office. Rather than just suctioning the fat, one first instills a large volume of fluid into the area from which the fat is to be removed. The solution contains three elements, saline, a local anesthetic, and epinephrine, to keep most of the small blood vessels in the area from bleeding. The tumescent technique obviates the need for general anesthetic, both because of the local anesthetic it contains and also because the fluid allows the fat to be removed much more easily, without damaging adjacent tissues and using a very small cannula to remove the fat. In my father's case, instillation of the fluid gave the additional advantage of making it easier to separate the fairly large piece of skin I would need for the graft from the underlying tissue without damaging it.

This part of the procedure actually takes the longest, since the patient must be prepped, then the fluid is instilled slowly. When I had finished, my father looked like someone with a bad case of mumps. He reached up to palpate his enormously engorged jowls.

"Will you hand me a mirror?" he asked my assistant, Virginia. "I can't imagine what I look like."

When he saw himself, he exclaimed, "I look like one of those little chameleons you and your brother used to keep, that could puff up their necks. Would you mind taking some pictures, Arthur? I want a record of the whole procedure."

After Virginia had taken a few pictures of him, I inserted a small cannula tip, no bigger than a wooden matchstick, and started the suction. When I had finished a few minutes later, my father's jawline was much sharper than it had been, although now, despite the small amount of swelling from the liposuction, his skin looked even slacker and more in need of a lift.

After numbing the skin on his neck, I again studied the photographs I had marked. Then I made identical marks on his neck to guide my incisions. I still felt a bit edgy. Naturally, I want every procedure I do to be successful for my patients, but it is equally true that I was particularly wound up due to the identity of my patient. Just as I picked up my scalpel and was about to begin the keyhole-shaped incision I would make, my father spoke up.

"How does it feel to be slitting your father's throat?" he asked.

Virginia giggled. "Don't make me laugh," I said, although I knew that he knew I was joking. I made a slow, steady, skin-deep incision down the midline of his neck, from his chin to just below his Adam's apple.

"Watch out you don't nick my carotid," he said, peering from under the sterile drape, as my gloved fingers slowly pulled the scalpel along his jawline. When I had finished, a scarlet T was beginning to form on his neck.

"More pictures, *please,* Arthur," he entreated.

"I don't usually take all these pictures for a patient's chart," I said.

"These aren't for my chart. They're for my own interest. This is a big deal for me, you know. I'm amazed by what you can do. I know I won't even be able to see a scar in a month or two, so I want a record."

"If you weren't my father, I'd be worried you were a litigious patient," I said with a laugh.

When I had dissected free the needed piece of skin, I put it aside in saline solution while I sutured the skin on his neck and tightened it around his reduced neck and lower jaw. It was like taking in a garment, only the cloth was in several layers, and I sewed the outer layer with thread thinner than a human hair in order to minimize scarring. As I finished this, the nurses prepped his lower leg. When he was ready, I laid the patch of neck skin over his wound, sewed it in place, and covered it with an airtight dressing to speed its healing. After we took several more pictures, my father was ready to go home.

A week later, he returned to the office so I could remove some of his stitches. Again he insisted on more pictures. Then, when he came in a week after that for the removal of the rest of the sutures, he wanted another full set.

I didn't see my parents for about a month after the operation, although my mother called several times to sing my praises and tell me how great my father looked. The next time we were all together was for Thanksgiving. By then, my father had had several months to heal. During dinner, I sneaked a look at him across the dinner table. He had always been a handsome man. Now, with his face and neck more defined, he looked like Jason Robards. It was an uncanny feeling to observe the change in my father's face and to realize it was I who had brought it about. We were all chatting in the living room when my father disappeared from the room and returned carrying two poster boards on which he had mounted and labeled the pictures of his operation.

I could see some of the nonmedical guests cringing as he passed his exhibit around the room.

"Ben, maybe some people don't like to look at things like that right after they've eaten," my mother suggested.

"But Sally, I'm so proud of him! Nobody today can even see a scar on my neck, so I wanted to show them how much cutting Arthur actually did."

My mother smiled and shrugged. I looked apologetically at the guests, but inside I was very pleased.

A few months later, I stopped by to visit my parents in Florida on the way home from a medical conference.

That evening, as my father and I sat watching the sun set, he pulled up his trouser leg. "Look," he said. "So far, no beard hair!"

We both laughed at the recollection of that day. For a moment, I felt swept up in the tide of my family. I was now in the second generation of doctors, and I was moving along. As my father had aged and given the stage to my ophthalmologist sister, Nancy, and me, I hoped I would one day be doing the same as one of my own children laid me down to perform the newest miracles of his or her generation of medicine upon my body.

INDEX

and skin color, 15–16, 134
and sun protection, 91, 92, 134,
136–37
and ultraviolet radiation, 136–37,
148
and vitiligo, 105
melanocytes, 15, 16, 17, 105
melanomas, 105, 129–35
ABCD system of, 141
age of onset, 140–41
biopsy for, 18, 138, 139–40, 141–
42
and immune system, 143
malignant, 129
metastasis of, 131, 140, 243
sites of, 141
spontaneous regression of, 143
statistics of, 140
treatment of, 143–44, 147–48
and ultraviolet radiation, 135–36,
140, 148–50
Merkel's disks, 21
metabolism, and aging, 93
methotrexate, 125, 126, 127
metronidazole, 228
micrografts, 193
mind-body connection, 184–89, 197,
206
minoxidil, 177–78, 189, 192
mnemoderma, 188
Mohs micrographic surgery, 89, 121,
143
molecular genetics, 122
moles, 17, 129
biopsies of, 145–47
dysplastic lesions, 151
and melanomas, 131, 141
monobenzylether of hydroquinone,
110
Montagu, Ashley, 2, 5
morphea, 58–73
and anti-hypertensive therapy, 70–
72
and collagen, 61, 62
diagnosis of, 61–64
recovery from, 72–73
and ticks, 60–61
treatment of, 63–72
see also scleroderma
multinucleated giant cells, 32
mycosis fungoides, 56

nasolabial folds, 231
necrolytic migratory erythema, 24
nervous system, and vitiligo, 105
neurosyphilis, 201, 203
nevocellular nevi (moles), 17, 129
New York Hospital-Cornell Medical
College, 155
night sweats, 37–38
nitrogen, liquid, 80, 232
nose, bulbous (rhinophyma), 227–30

oil of bergamot, 225
O'Malley, Dave (itching), 144–48
Ortega, Pilar (TB), 39–45
oxygen, and cell growth, 158
oxygen molecules, free radicals, 83–84
ozone layer, 134–35

parasitosis, delusions of, 200–201, 203
paresthesias, 201, 203
penicillamine, 63, 64–68
phenol peels, 214, 215
pheomelanin, 15
pheresis, 69–70
photopheresis, 69–70
phototherapy, 107, 109–10
pigment, 103, 107, 110
pimozide, 205–6
Pitanguy, Ivo, 209
placebo effect, 71
plant extracts, pharmaceutical, 110
Plaquenil, 51, 68, 69, 70
Potter, Jeff (xeroderma pigmentosum),
93–95
Pratt, Loretta (Balin), 163–64, 172–
73, 241
prednisone, 182
pregnancy, and PUVA therapy, 110–11
progesterone injections, 193–94, 197
protein chains, of collagen, 18
Prozac, 189
pruritus, see itching
psoralens, 110, 111, 225
psoriasis, 48, 114–20
causes of, 122, 123–24, 187
concomitant symptoms, 116, 120
eruptive, 124
guttate, 124
and immune system, 122–23
progression of, 122
pustular, 120–21, 124, 126, 127

About the Authors

Arthur K. Balin, M.D., Ph.D., F.A.C.P., is one of the foremost dermatologists in the country. Trained at the University of Pennsylvania School of Medicine, he has held academic appointments at Yale–New Haven Hospital, Cornell University Medical Center, the Rockefeller University, and Baylor University Medical Center. He is board certified in six medical specialties: internal medicine, dermatology, dermatopathology, geriatric medicine, Mohs micrographic surgery and cutaneous oncology, and dermatologic cosmetic surgery. He received a Ph.D. in biochemistry from the University of Pennsylvania. He is currently Clinical Professor of Dermatology and Research Professor of Pathology and Laboratory Medicine at the Allegheny University of the Health Sciences. He is executive director of the American Aging Association and Editor in Chief of the biomedical journal *Age*. In his clinical practice in Pennsylvania, he focuses on dermatology, Mohs micrographic surgery for skin cancer, and dermatologic cosmetic surgery. His research focuses on the basic biochemical mechanisms responsible for the aging process.

Loretta Pratt Balin, M.D., is a graduate of Barnard College and the Mount Sinai School of Medicine. She is board certified in dermatology and in internal medicine and was a fellow in investigative dermatology at the Rockefeller University. In her joint practice with her husband, she specializes in cosmetic dermatology and has a special interest in skin problems of women.

Marietta Whittlesey is a freelance writer specializing in medical topics.